Editor

Andrej Démuth

SPECTRUM SLOVAKIA Series
Volume 48

Cognitive, Semantic, and Evolutionary Aspects of Aesthetic and Moral Emotions

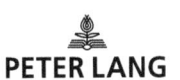

Bibliographic Information published by the Deutsche Nationalbibliothek
The Deutsche Nationalbibliothek lists this publication in the Deutsche Nationalbibliografie; detailed bibliographic data is available in the internet at http://dnb.d-nb.de.

Authors: Andrej Démuth, Slávka Démuthová, Renáta Kišoňová, Ľubomír Batka, Olexij M. Meteňkanyč

ISSN 2195-1845
ISBN 978-3-631-92569-0
ePDF 978-3-631-92570-6
ePub 978-3-631-92632-1
DOI 10.3726/b22295

ISBN 978-80-224-2075-4

© 2024 Peter Lang Group AG, Lausanne
Published by Peter Lang GmbH, Berlin, Germany

© VEDA, Publishing House of the Slovak Academy of Sciences
Bratislava 2024

All rights reserved.
Peter Lang – Berlin · Bruxelles · Chennai · Lausanne · New York · Oxford

All parts of this publication are protected by copyright. Any utilization outside the strict limits of the copyright law, without the permission of the publisher, is forbidden and liable to prosecution. This applies in particular to reproductions, translations, microfilming, and storage and processing in electronic retrieval systems.

www.peterlang.com

www.veda.sav.sk

This work was supported by the Slovak Research and Development Agency under the Contract no. APVV-19-0166. The authors also gratefully acknowledge the contribution of the Scientific Grant Agency of the Slovak Republic under the grant Vega no. 1/0120/22.

Photograph on the cover: Balthasar Permoser: Marsyas (ca. 1680–85). The MET, New York, Gallery 548.
Source: The Met. https://www.metmuseum.org/art/collection/search/211486

Contents

The Question Predetermines the Answer: Introduction as Foreshadowing of the Conclusion
Aesthetic and Moral Emotions
Andrej Démuth 7

Beauty
Historical Contexts and Contemporary Perspectives
Slávka Démuthová 15

Admiration and Disgust
Social and Moral Emotions of Admiration and Disgust
Renáta Kišoňová 65

Anger
The Awareness of Evil and the Defiant Decision to Take Justice into One's Own Hands
Andrej Démuth 95

Guilt
Persons in Web of Guilt. Guilt in Net of Interpretations
Ľubomír Batka 127

(In)justice
On the Indeterminacy of the Concept of (In)justice
Olexij M. Meteňkanyč 167

Outline of a Possible Mapping of Aesthetic and Moral Emotions
Summary or Conclusion?
Andrej Démuth 207

Notes on Contributors 221

The Question Predetermines the Answer: Introduction as Foreshadowing of the Conclusion
Aesthetic and Moral Emotions

Andrej Démuth

The five studies presented offer a somewhat unconventional analysis of aesthetic and moral emotions. This unconventionality arises not only from the approaches used but also from the chosen topics and terminology. The concept of moral emotions itself is relatively new, contributing to its ambiguity and controversy. Jonathan Haidt, in his famous article "The Moral Emotions" in the *Handbook of Affective Sciences*, defines moral emotions as those connected with social decision-making and actions aimed at the welfare of society as a whole, or at least the happiness of others besides the evaluator (Haidt, 2003). But are all moral emotions aimed at the welfare of others? And what does this welfare even mean? The definitions of aesthetic emotions are even more complex. There have been numerous attempts to define them or to discuss whether defining them is even necessary.[1] These are not new types of emotions or feelings. Moral emotions often include guilt, anger, shame, or injustice, while aesthetic emotions encompass beauty, admiration, or disgust. As works by Plato, Aristotle, Seneca, Lord Shaftesbury, Adam Smith, representatives of the Moral Sense School, Cambridge Platonists, Immanuel Kant, Max Scheler, and many others demonstrate, philosophers have long devoted attention to moral and aesthetic feelings. So what is unusual about the present reflections?

Firstly, there is a certain interdisciplinarity in their examination. The authors of the presented studies come from a wide range of disciplinary backgrounds. Slávka Démuthová is a psychologist, Renáta Kišoňová a philosopher, Andrej Démuth a philosopher and cognitive scientist, Luboš Batka a theologian, and Olexij M. Meteňkanyč a lawyer. The focal points of their work rely on slightly different explanatory frameworks, which also means different emphases on individual phenomena. Nevertheless, all authors believe in the need for a comprehensive interdisciplinary approach to their research. Through a series of joint meetings and consultations, they arrived at similar sets of questions to which they devote their attention.

The first is the representative selection of emotions and the need for terminological clarification. The authors recognize that

---

[1] See, for example, Menninghaus, et al. (2019), Skov, Nadal (2020), Menninghaus et al. (2020), Démuth, Démuthová (2023).

both aesthetic and moral emotions encompass a wide range of different perceptions, feelings, emotions, and emotional states. Many of these are entirely distinct, yet some are similar and often mixed, both in terms of experience and terminology. Therefore, they primarily attempt to (a) define the basic concepts of selected moral/aesthetic intentional objects, feelings, experiences, and emotions (in the aesthetic realm, e.g., beauty; at the intersection of aesthetic and moral emotions, admiration and disgust; and in the realm of moral experiences, feelings of injustice, anger, and guilt). A common feature of their investigations is that these concepts are understood as central overarching terms that capture a wide (convex) area of diverse perceptions, feelings, emotions, and states. Through conceptual analysis of the individual connotations of the examined terms (for instance: Démuthová, 2023), they aim to establish the basic qualitative and semantic domains of these terms, hoping to delineate the fundamental horizontal structure of aesthetic and moral states (from defining intentional objects, through feelings and experiences to complex emotions and their combinations), as well as their vertical (hierarchical) structure (from the most basic to the most significant). Similar mapping of basic semantic levels is also offered by examining individual antonyms or opposites of the given terms, which indicate various possible semantic levels of how the terms are used and what they actually denote in different contexts. It turns out that even basic overarching terms are not unambiguous but rather multidimensional, and thus, even the basic emotions and terms used to denote them may not have clear opposites but instead possess a whole group of possible opposing feelings and states, depending on the qualitative dimension being evaluated.

Despite the diversity of individual perceptions, feelings, emotions, and emotional states, and the effort to preserve this diversity, the common feature of the presented chapters is (b) the attempt to explain the semantic relationships between the examined terms and concepts (their placement within the semantic space of individual aesthetic and moral concepts). Based on this, they aim to point out semantic similarities and proximities within individual aesthetic emotions, within moral emotions, and between aesthetic and moral emotions. They are interested in which emotions are close to which and why.

A characteristic feature of the presented texts is the analysis of subjective experience associated with the above-selected aesthetic and moral emotions (what we experience and how we describe experiencing a particular emotion from a first-person perspective). The authors often use various versions of phenomenological and hermeneutic-existential analysis, focusing not only on the description of the given experience with a particular emotion but also on what that experience means for the individual and how it is understood. This brings us to another common feature of the presented studies – their evolutionary perspective.

The authors often reflect on the role these emotional states play not only from the perspective of individuals but also from the perspective of the entire species they represent. They consider why a given emotional state exists, what evolutionary role it has played, and whether it still plays a role. Is the emotion still necessary for humans? From a biological perspective, one can consider the phylogenetic development of perceiving a given emotion and its roles for the species, as well as the ontogenetic development of our ability to feel these emotions. Are we born with the ability to perceive beauty, disgust, anger, guilt, and injustice, or do we acquire these abilities gradually? Is their content consistent throughout life, or does it undergo significant changes?

Part of the authors also explore the neurobiological foundations or correlates of the given emotional experience. They examine neuroscientific research related to aesthetic and moral emotions, analyzing their neuronal correlates, determinants, and potential disorders (especially of the reward system and limbic system) and their interconnections. Through literature review and partial own research, they attempt to find correlations between subjective experience and objective neuronal data (brain activity and neuronal correlates of the given emotion or experience) or psychological manifestations. They are interested in: what are the neuronal representations of aesthetic and moral emotions? Do they share any common areas of neuronal activity? If so, what does this mean?

The authors of the chapters are primarily humanities-oriented scholars; thus, their main interest is aligning the interpretation of aesthetic and moral emotions from a first-person perspective with current neuroscientific research on the mechanisms and processes of aesthetic and moral emotions. They attempt to create a (as comprehensive as possible) integrated concept of aesthetic and moral emotions that considers both the subjective perception of these emotional states and the objective description of these phenomena from a societal or current cognitively oriented research perspective.

A common feature of the individually studied emotional states is not only that they are consciously experienced but also that they motivate us to a specific type of behavior. Therefore, the authors consider selected emotions not only individually but also examine them in the context of their similarities and similarities. A typical feature of some feelings, for instance, is that we subjectively experience them as good or pleasant (e.g., beauty, admiration). Others, on the contrary, are perceived with displeasure, evoke distinctly unpleasant feelings, and urge us to change and eliminate the given state (disgust, anger, guilt, injustice). This similar or identical experience of different emotions is caused not only by the similarity of the compositions and levels of involved neuromodulators (predominantly dopamine for positive ones, serotonin, and norepinephrine for negative ones), the activity of common neuroanatomical and neurophysiological structures (reward circuit) and processes, but primarily by the similar function they play in our lives and the tasks they pose for us. It is therefore understandable that one of the aims of the presented research was to consider the mutual connection between aesthetic and moral emotions (hoping to uncover basic cognitive aspects or patterns of both types of emotions, documenting universal or culturally conditioned evaluations of perception and cognitive judgments), their similarities, differences, or possible causal connections. In everyday language, we often interchange the terms "beautiful and good", "ugly and bad[2] – although they should refer to seemingly entirely different qualities of perceived phenomena. Is it possible to strictly separate both groups of emotions, or is it possible that, for example, beauty is good? Is goodness beautiful? Is it just a matter of confusing terms due to linguistic ignorance or metaphorical language, or does this confusion stem from deeper, common neuronal or experiential reasons?

---

[2] For example, when we say that a painting is well or beautifully done, or conversely, that an action was not nice or good (thus it was ugly or bad).

The aim of the presented chapters is to synthesize research findings into (as much as possible) a unified concept of aesthetic and moral emotions. The collective monograph is the result of a long-term project titled *"Analysis of the Conceptual and Qualitative Domains of Aesthetic and Moral Emotions"*,[3] conducted between 2020 and 2024 at Comenius University in Bratislava and the University of St Cyril and Methodius in Trnava. It represents a summary output of a series of partial studies.[4] The entire project included systematic research on aesthetic and moral emotions – their selected examples as psychosomatic phenomena, from a first-person perspective with a focus on hermeneutic-phenomenological-existential analysis of the basic elements, structure, and significance of this type of emotions in human experience. Whether this research has fulfilled its goals (or possibly prompts the reader to deeper contemplation about emotions, or even moves them to some action) is left to the judgment of the reader.

References

Démuth, A. (2024a). *Anger as A/Moral Emotion*. Peter Lang.

Démuth, A. (2024b). O hneve, alebo čo ponúka Heideggerova filozofia afektivity. [On Anger, or What Heidegger's Philosophy of Affectivity Offers]. *Filozofický časopis.* 72(3), 415–429.

Démuth, A., and Démuthová, S. (2023). A Conceptual and Semantic Analysis of the Qualitative Domains of Aesthetic and Moral Motions: An Introduction. In: Démuth, A. and Démuthová, S. (eds.). *A Conceptual and Semantic Analysis of the Qualitative Domains of Aesthetic and Moral Emotions.* (pp. 7–38), Peter Lang Verlag.

Démuth. A., Démuthová, S., and Keçeli, Y. (2022). A Semantic Analysis of the Concept of Beauty (Güzellik) in Turkish Language: Mapping the Semantic Domains. *Frontiers in communication* 7:797316. doi: 10.3389/fcomm.2022.797316

---

[3] This work was supported by the Slovak Research and Development Agency under the Contract no. APVV-19-0166, and by the the Scientific Grant Agency of the Slovak Republic under the Contract no. 1/0120/22.

[4] This book was preceded by the publication of an entire series of scientific studies and monographs, such as those by Démuth, A. Démuthová (2023), Démuth (2024), and Démuthová, Kišoňová, and Démuth (2024a), and studies by Démuth (2004b) and Démuth, Démuthová, Keceli (2022).

Démuthová, S. (2023). The Possibilities of Studying Connotations of the Term "Beauty" in a Natural Language In: A. Démuth, S. Démuthová, (eds.) *A Conceptual and Semantic Analysis of the Qualitative Domains of Aesthetic and Moral Emotions: An Introduction.* (pp. 57–80), Peter Lang,

Démuthová, S., Kišoňová, R., and Démuth, A. (2024). *Pojem krása. Krása ako estetická emócia.* [The Concept of Beauty: Beauty as an Aesthetic Emotion]. Veda.

Haidt, J. (2003). The Moral Emotions. In Davidson, Richard, Scherer, Klaus, and Goldsmith, H. (eds.). *Handbook of Affective Sciences.* Oxford University Press.

Menninghaus, W., Wagner, V., Wassiliwizky, E., Schindler, I., Hanich, J., Jacobsen, T., and Koelsch, S. (2019). What are aesthetic emotions?. *Psychological review, 126*(2), 171–195. https://doi.org/10.1037/rev0000135.

Menninghaus, W., Schindler, I., Wagner, V., Wassiliwizky, E., Hanich, J., Jacobsen, T., and Koelsch, S. (2020). Aesthetic emotions are a key factor in aesthetic evaluation: Reply to Skov and Nadal (2020). *Psychological review, 127*(4), 650–654. https://doi.org/10.1037/rev0000213

Skov, M., and Nadal, M. (2020). There are no aesthetic emotions: Comment on Menninghaus et al. (2019). *Psychological review, 127*(4), 640–649. https://doi.org/10.1037/rev0000187

Beauty
Historical Contexts
and Contemporary Perspectives

Slávka Démuthová

The beautiful is a manifestation of secret laws of nature which – without its appearance – would have remained hidden from us forever.

Johann Wolfgang von Goethe
Maxims and reflections, No. 183

Despite the fact that beauty belongs to one of the most influential concepts shaping both personal and societal attitudes (including values, desires, attitudes, preferences, etc.), it seems to lack a coherent and universally accepted definition. On one hand, scientific attempts to delineate this concept have been numerous; on the other hand, many assert that the understanding of beauty is highly subjective and individual (de gustibus non disputandum, beauty is in the eye of the beholder), leading to the conclusion that a unified concept of beauty does not exist. Despite these challenges, the exploration of beauty has captivated attention for centuries and remains a subject of inquiry across various academic disciplines. The fact remains that, despite the long-standing interest in its essence, a universal definition of beauty is still elusive, prompting continual investigation by scholars. From the research conducted thus far, it is evident that a comprehensive understanding of what beauty entails necessitates consideration of multiple contexts and dimensions. Primarily, historical examination of the concept of beauty proves beneficial in two contexts: the first involves uncovering historical perspectives on beauty (i.e., the development of the understanding and perception of beauty over time), and the second aims to identify the mechanisms behind the perception and evaluation of beauty as an evolutionarily conditioned tendency to perceive and evaluate certain objects as beautiful. Beyond this universal "macro level", it is also crucial to acknowledge that the understanding of beauty is influenced by numerous factors with a smaller scope ("micro level"), yet these factors equally shape the comprehension of the concept. These factors include, for instance, language, an individual's current mood; the context in which beauty is assessed; media influences, age, gender, and many others. Through the examination of each of these factors, it is possible to identify the diversity of beauty preferences.

Historical Contexts

Focusing on the European cultural environment and Western civilization, it is evident that the concept of beauty significantly stems from philosophical concepts presented throughout history. In interpreting the notion of beauty, it is essential to consider the "traditional" components and characteristics of beautiful objects defined as early as antiquity (such as proportion, symmetry, etc.), the more recent applications of empirically justifiable rules emphasized during the Renaissance, and the findings of current research exploring correlations between external signs of beauty and the hidden parameters of physical fitness in organisms. A comprehensive overview of the history of the understanding of beauty cannot be provided within this limited scope. Instead, the aim of this subchapter is to draw attention to how taste, the concept of beauty, and attractiveness are determined by historical influences. These influences are linked to geographical, cultural, and religious contexts, as well as the dominant philosophical concepts of each period.

Prehistoric Period

In the absence of written records documenting the modes of thought and perspectives on the issue of beauty, our exploration of this concept and human preferences relies predominantly on the interpretation of human artifacts. As with any interpretation, this approach carries a high risk of misinterpretation. For instance, experts often speculate that if the practical function of an object, or its part, or a specific design is unclear, it might be assumed to serve an aesthetic purpose. According to Haselberger, an artistic object is one that was produced with the intention that it be aesthetically pleasing and not merely pragmatically functional (Haselberger, 1961). This definition undoubtedly has merit; however, the challenge lies in estimating from a contemporary perspective what was considered "aesthetically pleasing" to our ancestors and understanding the various pragmatic functions - hidden to us - that these objects might have had. We can only speculate that a drawing on clothing or an engraving on a weapon was intended to beautify the object, and we might infer the aesthetic preferences of its creator. Yet, we cannot be certain whether the drawing on the clothing did not indicate tribal affiliation or whether the engraving on the weapon hadn´t a religious function, such as protecting the owner from the spirits of the animals killed. Although the painting of garments, pots, or dwellings is regarded as evidence of early art, we cannot be sure that this was indeed the case. If we accept the hypothesis that the oldest discovered cave paintings date back more than 64,800 years (Hoffmann et al., 2018), it highlights the vast expanse of history regarding the perception and depiction of beauty that is currently relegated to conjecture and speculation.

Antiquity

Even from relatively recent history (in comparison to the vast length of history involving the creation of potential art), there are relatively few records that shed light on how our ancestors perceived beauty and what they understood by this concept. However, it is possible to assert with certainty that these views have changed over time, as evidenced by several approaches identifiable in antiquity.

In earlier periods (in the 5th century BCE), Athenian sophists held a relatively narrow view of beauty, associating it with objects that are pleasant to see or hear. This specification was natural for sensualists; moreover, its advantage was that it better defined the concept of beauty by distinguishing it from goodness (Tatarkiewicz, 1980). Goodness (as well as other values like correctness and appropriateness) has often been historically associated with beauty (e.g., the Delphic maxim "what is right is beautiful") (Eco, 2005), and this connection was characteristic of various concepts developed during antiquity. Perhaps the most influential aesthetic ideal of ancient Greece is kalokagathia. The etymology of the word (kalos + agathos) indicates that it is a combination of beauty (as an external quality) and goodness (as an internal quality). In ancient thought, a beautiful person is one who is both attractive and good. Beauty and goodness form a unity – this connection persists in many ways to this day and can be identified in well-known stereotypes (e.g., the "what is beautiful is good" stereotype – Dion et al., 1972) and cognitive biases (e.g., the "halo effect" – Nisbett & Wilson, 1977) described primarily in social psychology.

Socrates distinguished three types of beauty: ideal beauty, which reflects nature; spiritual beauty, which captures the soul through appearance; and useful beauty, whose significance lies in its purpose (Eco, 2005). In contrast, according to Plato, true beauty is only one and universally valid; it is one of the highest ideals (Lloyd, 2010). Within this idealistic philosophical framework, it can be explained that the reason for the existence of multiple kinds and variants of beauty in the world is that they are merely reflections of ideal beauty, whose existence is independent of the object to which it is attached. Carriers of beauty – objects we label as beautiful – are merely incidental reflections of true beauty, which is not bound to any perceivable object. Art, therefore, is only a false copy of true beauty. According to Plato, what best captures the essence of beauty is harmony and proportion, represented, for example, by the beauty of geometric forms (Eco, 2005) and the beauty of law (Platón, 1979).

Although deriving an understanding of beauty from artistic works has its pitfalls (as previously described), it is evident that many ancient works were created to respect or even represent contemporary ideals of beauty. Buildings were constructed using aesthetic principles (e.g., the golden ratio, symmetry, the Pythagorean scale, etc.), musical works were composed based on numerical relationships to be pleasant and beautiful, and sculptors applied principles of correct proportions. Many ancient ideals were revived in later periods across various fields of art and science – for example, in the form of returns to their ideas (e.g., in philosophy and art during the Middle Ages through Neoplatonism – Dürrigl, 2002) or even in 21st-century plastic surgery (the golden ratio as an ideal of facial proportions – Hwang & Park, 2021).

Medieval Period

During the medieval period, Plato's ideas of beauty and goodness became significantly Christianized. Beauty was primarily associated with qualities such as moderation, modesty, and other virtues, and it was perceived mainly in the context of what can be termed "inner beauty," meaning the beauty of the soul. Preoccupation with external beauty was considered as vanity, lust, and corruption of the body (Dürrigl, 2002). However, it would be a mistake to assume that all medieval approaches to beauty shared the idea of Neoplatonism in this form. Although the dualism of soul and body was characteristic of the medieval period, this dualism did not always set these two components in opposition within the context of beauty and goodness. A significant portion of the medieval period was influenced by the Augustinian idea that both the body and the soul are good, but the body is handicapped compared to the soul due to its mortality and the temporality of its existence. Thus, the appreciation of external, physical beauty was often coupled with an awareness of its transience. As Boethius wrote, external beauty is as fleeting as spring flowers (Boëthius, 1929). Many mystical works, however, did not avoid depicting external beauty and often made it a central motif. In the context of medieval thought, beauty becomes visible and active primarily when the soul "illuminates" the body in harmony with the object (Dürrigl, 2002).

In medieval approaches (especially in Latin medieval thought), one can also identify an Aristotelian objectifying and rationalizing approach. This approach was not primarily based on proportions and mathematics when depicting the human body (since corporeality was subordinate to spiritual beauty), but it employed a Pythagorean-proportional approach in defining moral beauty. A deeper emphasis on the attribute of proportion is evident in the conception of Thomas Aquinas, who highlighted three aesthetic qualities of an object: integritas (wholeness), proportio (proportion), and claritas (clarity) (Démuthová et al., 2024).

In attempting to understand the medieval concept of beauty from a modern perspective, a fundamental issue is the lack of clear distinction in the Middle Ages between beauty, utility, and goodness (similarly to how in antiquity there was no strict boundary between goodness and beauty). Moral and aesthetic reactions to things were unified and intertwined. Hence, many saints were depicted not only as devout, virtuous, good, and chaste but also as beautiful (Dürrigl, 2002). Another issue is that many views on the Middle Ages are overly simplistic – this period is often collectively labeled as the "Dark Ages", even though it was certainly not dark throughout and in all aspects (Rahman, 2003). In this context, Pradier (2022) highlighted several intellectual currents related to the understanding of beauty that emerged in the medieval period. He identified three tensions leading to three turning points: (1) the categorical distinction between beauty and appropriateness (St. Augustine of Hippo and St. Isidore of Seville, who raise this issue in the Latin patristic tradition); (2) the contrast between aesthetic judgment based on functional satisfaction and judgment based on the free and pure appearance of the object (St. Basil the Great); and 3) the debate on the practical value of the aesthetic stance through the texts of Hugh of St. Victor, St. Bernard of Clairvaux, and Suger of St. Denis. Pradier's conclusions reveal the "irreducible aesthetic value of functional beauty in the medieval period and the extraordinary difficulties in accommodating a free and autonomous notion of beauty, as well as the practical benefits of its everyday treatment. In fact, the consideration of free beauty as a good in itself persists in medieval thought, which is important not only for the History of Philosophy but also for contemporary concerns shared by Philosophy of Religion and Aesthetics about the role of sensitive beauty in the life of human being" (Pradier, 2022, 1). It should be noted that several ideas presented in the Middle Ages resonated in later periods as well. Aquinas's view that beauty and goodness are logically distinct and the notion that beauty is a transcendental property, which reveals itself in relation to the knowing subject, were, for instance, significant contributions toward humanism (Dürrigl, 2002).

Renaissance

The principles of beauty during the Renaissance period can be identified in numerous works by painters (such as Piero della Francesca), mathematicians (Luca Pacioli), architects (Leon Battista Alberti), philosophers (Marsilio Ficino), and polymaths (Leonardo da Vinci). Renaissance ideas were inspired by the tenets of humanism, with a clear effort to revive and emulate the literature and art of the ancient Greeks and Romans. Artists began to reproduce classical images, copying ancient sculptures – art during this period was significantly influenced by this background (Haughton, 2004). One of the leading humanists, Marcus Marulus Spalatensis, in his extensive work Repertorium, written around 1500, cites Plato under the entry "Bonum" with the phrase "Pulchritudo est summi bonum splendor" (beauty is the splendor of the highest good); in the semantic sense of "beautiful", imaginary features of perfection and nobility often play a role (Dürrigl, 2002).

Similarly to antiquity, during the Renaissance, the evaluation of beauty and artistic works to some extent required that objects accurately correspond to reality and be proportionately expressed. The study of beauty focused on identifying fixed, objectifiable, scientifically justified rules; beautiful objects were then those that adhered to the laws of perspective, anatomy, the physiological science of movement, respecting the golden ratio, and free from contradictions with a high degree of harmony, whether in the arrangement of colors, qualities, or proportions (Démuthová et al., 2024). The effort to create art that would produce physically perfect images arising from professional expectations, the artist's ambitions, and his developing skills often resulted in a tendency to avoid realistic interpretation and instead emphasize primarily the positive attributes of objects (Haughton, 2004).

Symmetry, harmony, proportion, and many other canons of beauty were important characteristics of the Renaissance period; however (as can be seen within the diversity of human creativity and taste), they were not the only ones. Alongside the mainstream preferences, parallel trends emerged that diverged from the dominant views. An example of this is the presence of tendencies to focus on dynamic, restless beauty that surprises the observer. Anticipated principles were disrupted or denied, introducing into art and other fields related to the presentation of beauty a need to capture the contemporary "spirit" of the time or moment. These trends can be simplified and associated with the currents of classicism, mannerism, baroque, or rococo. In connection with beauty, themes such as grace, elegance, melancholy, ingenuity, and agudeza appeared (Eco, 2005). Despite the dynamic development of opinions on beauty and aesthetic taste during the Renaissance, Neoplatonic philosophical concepts survived into the modern era.

Modern Era

The burgeoning of education, technological progress, and the availability of information have brought numerous changes to society, including a variability of perspectives and opinions. If it was difficult to generalize views on beauty in previous periods, it is essentially impossible in the modern era. Even a brief overview of the main ideas would be unfeasible in such a limited space. Therefore, only selected tendencies can be outlined to illustrate how perspectives on beauty have changed throughout history.

An important momentum of the Modern Era in relation to the understanding of beauty was the effort to identify the reasons for the emergence of modern aesthetic theory. In this field, Kant's works on aesthetics, particularly *"Critique of Judgment"*, *"Critique of Pure Reason"*, and *"Critique of Practical Reason"*, proved to be crucial (Bowie, 2003). Démuth provided interesting insights in this regard – he analyzed Hume's concept of the standardization of tastes, Reid's aesthetic realism, and Kant's mathematical standardization. According to Démuth, for Hume, beauty relates to transcending the standard, that is, what most observers perceive as unusual, pleasing, and positively exceptional. In Thomas Reid's mathematization of objects, beauty is a real quality of the object (we perceive objects, not feelings). Beauty does not reside in the eye of the beholder but in the object itself – its parameters can be measured and mathematically analyzed. An aesthetic judgment is therefore possible only based on an understanding of the object. Kant's approach may seem paradoxical in this context (since, according to him, an aesthetic judgment involves reflective judgment, which is devoid of concepts and intellectual purposes), yet principles for forming an aesthetic evaluation can be derived from it. The creation of the idea of a beauty norm occurs through an unconscious mathematical calculation based on experience. Through perception and analysis of objects, we create a certain prototype, a model of a given class of objects, which results from averaging experiences. The closer a particular assessed object is to such a prototype, the more beautiful it is judged to be. While Hume prefers the median in evaluating the beauty of an object, Kant considers the arithmetic mean, taking into account the frequency of individual experiences. This, then, justifies the need to refine taste by frequently encountering beautiful objects (Démuth, 2016).

During the Modern Era, particularly in German idealist philosophy (Démuth, Rušinová, 2019), a multitude of philosophers and artists expressed themselves on the issue of beauty – Schiller believed that beauty is "thus nothing less than freedom in appearance" (Schiller, 1943, XXVI, p. 183, Schiller, 1793/2003, p. 152); Schlegel defines "beauty" as "what is at once charming and sublime, and for Schelling the sublime is sublime only to the extent that it is beautiful; for Hegel, the "beauty" of artworks is a function of the profundity of the "inner truth of their content and thought" (Kirwan, 2023, p. 23). For Lyotard, beauty was not serious enough – it is a mere matter of taste, addressing itself to "the 'common sense' of a shared pleasure"; Levinson stresses, that when perceiving beauty, it is not a matter of merely passive sensation but rather an active enjoyment (Kirwan, 2023). Bascom presented an intriguing perspective in this regard – he plainly stated that beauty is not the "exclusive object" of the fine arts (Bascom, 1867).

The exploration of beauty did indeed expand into many fields during the Modern Era. Beauty has gradually become a subject of interest not only in philosophy, art, and mathematics but in almost all scientific fields. Biology (Vaidyanathan et al., 2023), aesthetics (Dietrich & Knieper, 2022), psychology (Rhodes, 2006), neurology (Yang et al., 2022), architecture (Coburn et al., 2017), medicine (Riji, 2006), design (Shi et al., 2021), linguistics (Menninghaus et al., 2019)... all engage with the concept of beauty. The study of beauty is currently a highly developed area of research and the fascination with beauty is evident not only in science but also in everyday life. The modern era is even characterized by its "age of beauty", where beauty often takes precedence over other attributes such as functionality (fashion) or even health (plastic surgery, skin whitening, etc.). In this regard, philosopher and theologian Zanchi in his book "*La bellezza complice*" (Zanchi, 2020) proposes that we live in the era of the "omnipresence of beauty, but, of course, of apparent beauty; that of consumerism; that which is manipulated, masked; that of cosmetic, which hides and clouds the truth. Beauty has come out 'from the supernatural room' of its transcendent dimension and, everyday, becoming trivialized; it has become an instrument and accomplice of concealment. It could be said that she has denied herself, losing her true essence, her relationship with the soul, with goodness, with the purity of the 'knight without a sword" who carries the heart of a good man" (Musicco Nombela, 2024, p. 15). A significant element that influences views on beauty, alongside considerable plurality, is globalization. Amid countless notions of what constitutes beauty, there is a trend of adopting tastes from often very distant backgrounds, whether geographically or culturally. Globalization, particularly through high individual mobility and the global influence of media and communication networks, has led to the blending of previously separate and distinct tendencies. Despite intensive and long-standing research into the study of beauty, as well as lay interest in the topic, a unified definition of beauty still does not exist. Its attributes their significance, the perception of beauty, or its evaluation, and the factors that influence these processes, as well as the strength of their determination, remain sources of many questions.

Historical perspectives have presented numerous views on beauty. Some were temporary, while others persisted or periodically reemerged throughout history. Interestingly, many principles preferred during the historical study of beauty have proven to be more than mere trends of their time. The validity of several historical views and approaches to beauty has been confirmed through modern empirical research. It appears that historically formulated views on beauty may not be merely manifestations of abstract ideas shaped by the cultural environment in which they were created but pointed to key features of beautiful objects, such as those based on fundamental biological principles (objectifying the concept of beauty) and carrying essential, evolutionarily significant characteristics.

Evolutionary Contexts

Contemporary evolutionary psychology proves that the assessment of objects, situations or phenomena as beautiful occurs because they point to a biologically desirable characteristic for the existence of that organism (Démuth, 2019 – what is beautiful is perceived as such because it is healthy, high-quality, resilient, etc.). This can be observed in various contexts of studying beauty and beautiful objects, most intensely in relation to the human body and face, however, though the evolutionary basis for the preference of certain traits can also be identified in inanimate objects.

The Beautiful Body

A cross-section of the history of figurative art as a source of information on the conception of the beauty of the human body might seem confusing at first glance – the Paleolithic Venus of Dolní Věstonice (Vandiver et al., 1989) is vastly different from the Twiggy cult of the 1960s (Montgomery Sklar, 2015). Even considering the possibility that depictions of human figures in prehistoric times may not necessarily represent an ideal of beauty but were specifically portrayed for other reasons (religious, symbolic, etc.), the forms that painters or sculptors later presented and themselves labeled as beautiful bodies varied significantly throughout history. These facts suggest almost exclusive determination by cultural, temporal, individual, and other preferences, indicating a highly subjective, variable, and elusive concept of the beauty of the human body. On the other hand, it is interesting to observe that, although the specific forms of what is considered a beautiful human figure may have changed over time and geographic space, attention was mostly focused on the same features – in women, primarily the hips, waist, and breasts; in men, the shoulders and chest, or the upper body. Certain body parts or traits attract more attention than others and appear to be key for the final assessment of attractiveness. This insight has led to attempts to objectify the beauty of the human figure and inspired scientists to numerous studies.

The entire era of specific research focused on objectifying the characteristics of beautiful male and female bodies across cultures has yielded significant results. Despite some variability in preferences when selecting a beautiful figure, it appears that in evolutionarily significant situations (a typical example being mate selection), the characteristics of a beautiful body are relatively universal. Attention is drawn to certain body parts that signal an individual's genetic quality as well as their current health and fitness. In evaluating the beauty of the female body, proportions are likely the most important, specifically the waist-to-hip ratio (WHR). Studies have found that men consider a WHR close to 0.7 to be the most attractive across cultures (Dixson et al., 2010), with this ratio holding even amidst varying preferences for the optimal weight of a woman (Sugiyama, 2004). The evolutionary significance of this preference spans several areas: a narrow waist in a woman signals youth, and thus the potential to be a suitable partner. It is also one of the few visible signs indicating that a woman is not currently pregnant (ergo not momentarily infertile and not long-term encumbered with the care of another's offspring) (Singh, 1993). A wide pelvis, on the other hand, indicates suitable fat storage necessary for the nourishment of the fetus, particularly for the healthy development of the baby's brain (Lassek & Gaulin, 2008). Fat storage in the hips is not associated with health risks as it is in the waist area. A larger hip circumference compared to the waist is also an indicator that during pregnancy, there will be enough room for fetal growth and that the birth canal will be sufficiently wide for an uncomplicated delivery. A wide pelvis also helps maintain stability while walking, especially during pregnancy and lactation (Pawłowski, 2001). Correlational studies have also shown that WHR values close to 0.7 are closely associated with optimal hormone levels, lower incidences of miscarriages (Hahn et al., 2014; Felisbino-Mendes et al., 2014), and lower rates of cardiovascular diseases, diabetes, and cancer (Singh & Singh, 2011; World Health Organization: WHO, 2008). It is evident that the presence of specific body characteristics, which people subjectively evaluate as beautiful, reflects objective qualities – indicators of the health of the individual and woman´s ability to conceive, carry, give birth to, nurture, and raise offspring.

The beautiful male body has also been the subject of numerous studies. Similar to the identification of a WHR of 0.7 as attractive in women, men's WHR represents a significant characteristic. For women, an attractive WHR in men is slightly higher, with the most preferred value being around 0.9 (Singh, 1995). However, in evaluating the beauty of the male body, other characteristics also play a role – particularly the width of the shoulders and the "robustness" of the upper body (Salusso-Deonier et al., 1993), expressed either by the waist-to-shoulder ratio (WSR) with a value of 0.6 (Dixson et al., 2003) or the waist-to-chest ratio (WCR) (Maisey et al., 1999). Broad shoulders and strength associated with pronounced upper body musculature indicate physical strength, which provides an advantage in combat and direct physical confrontation with rivals, whether in the struggle for survival or competition for a mate. These characteristics prove to be reliable indicators for women seeking healthy men with good genes and potentially successful in survival challenges. Men with an optimal WHR value are not only optimally built for combat with competitors but are also genuinely healthier, less frequently suffering from prostate cancer (Jackson et al., 2010), gallbladder, and bile duct cancer (Zhang et al., 2005), and have better cholesterol levels and blood pressure (Katsilambros et al., 1993). WHR is even shown to be a more important indicator of overall health than the more commonly used BMI index (Tambe et al., 2010) or waist circumference (Hubbard et al., 2004). Besides body composition, other masculine traits play a role in attractiveness evaluations, such as body hair as a significant indicator of sexual maturity (Dixson et al., 2003). Additional traits related to facial features are described in the following subchapters.

The Beautiful Face

If there have been historical scientific efforts to objectify the human body, the face has inspired scientists to engage in even more intense research. The face holds a unique significance as an object of human perception. Through the face, one can recognize a familiar person, estimate the age of an unfamiliar individual, discern their current emotional state, and gauge their awareness of the surrounding environment. The ability to see another person's face facilitates, supplements, and refines the content of verbal communication, and it can even replace this type of communication entirely. The perception of another person's face also plays a significant role in the survival of the individual at its most fundamental biological level. It enables the identification of a potential reproductive partner (through recognizing the gender of the other individual), their fertility (through age estimation), genetic potential and long-term health (e.g., by evaluating facial symmetry and averageness), current health status (skin coloration and quality), and even the identification of traits that suggest personality compatibility in a relationship (personality and intellect estimation, etc.). Thus, the face, in its complexity, serves as an essential indicator of health, resilience, reproductive value, and the riskiness of the individual, as well as other information crucial for the preservation of the individual and their genes.

The exceptional nature of facial perception was so vital in phylogenesis that the mechanisms of receiving, processing, and evaluating information about human faces became automated (face evaluation occurs without conscious effort) and influence our behavior even at an unconscious level (much of the information we receive and evaluate from faces is not directly accessible to conscious analysis) (Hung et al., 2016). Many of these mechanisms exhibit signs of being innate. Additionally, neuroanatomical studies have shown that a specific neural network in the brain has developed to handle (often uniquely and exclusively) the processing of face-related stimuli. It appears that the information obtained from faces has been (and continues to be) so critical for individual survival that it has led to the development of functional, anatomical, and systemic specializations in the brain tailored to process this type of data. These specialized areas are further connected to key systems that modify human behavior, particularly the reward systems and the systems responsible for emitting emotions (Pitcher et al., 2011).

The importance of the human face is reflected in the numerous characteristics identified as universal keys for discerning the essential traits of its bearer. In the context of the aforementioned evolutionary pressures, these traits are also perceived (almost universally) as beautiful. Among the most significant are symmetry, averageness, the presence of sexually dimorphic features, and neoteny.

Symmetry is a characteristic identified in relation to beautiful objects since ancient times. Aristotle described orderliness and symmetry as primary forms associated with beauty (Aristotle, 2004). Cicero characterized a beautiful body as symmetrical (Cicero, 1971), and Plotinus asserted that beautiful things are inherently symmetrical (Plotinus, 2016). However, it is necessary to note that in antiquity (and later during the Renaissance by figures such as Leonardo da Vinci, Albrecht Dürer, and Leon Battista Alberti), the concept of symmetry was understood more broadly than it is today (Etcoff, 1999). In contemporary usage, symmetry is primarily expressed as the congruence (usually along the central axis or plane of an object), identicality, or sameness of two parts of an object that lie on opposite sides of such an axis/plane. More generally, an object is called symmetrical if there exists a transformation that leaves the object as a whole unchanged (Vrábel, 2005). From an evolutionary perspective, symmetry is an indication of an organism's developmental stability (Simmons et al., 2004; Danescu et al., 2021; Gangestad, 2022, etc.). Deviations from symmetry result from an organism's failure to cope with various adverse environmental (e.g., climate, pollution, malnutrition, parasitism – Grammer & Thornhill, 1994; Agnew & Koella, 1997) or genetic (e.g., inbreeding, mutations – Møller, 1997) factors during ontogeny. Research has shown that women with more asymmetrical faces exhibited poorer resilience to physical stress, while men displayed higher levels of depression and emotional instability (Shackelford & Larsen, 1997). Asymmetry in men is significantly associated with lifelong health handicaps (Møller, 1990) and reduced fertility (Manning et al., 1998). Moreover, organismal symmetry correlates with growth and survival indices (Livshits & Kobyliansky, 1994; Little et al., 2008), potential (Jasienska et al., 2006) and actual fertility, and age-dependent fecundity (Møller et al., 1995) in women.

The concept of averageness refers to the principle of familiarity – familiar things evoke positive feelings in us, while the unknown trigger caution, fear (Cao et al., 2011), and even hostility. For an organism striving for survival, an unfamiliar object or organism represents a potential source of danger. Therefore, its presence heightens vigilance, caution, tension, and readiness to defend or escape when necessary. Fear of the unknown or xenophobia is considered a fundamental fear (Carleton, 2016). Based on this mechanism, an object that we encounter more frequently and does not pose a threat to us elicits more positive reactions than something unfamiliar or unusual. An average face is the result of our experience with human faces – it represents a kind of prototype, an average. Research is conducted in various types of societies and individuals from different religions, cultures, and levels of development; multicultural and isolated communities indeed indicate that in every community, an average face is rated as more attractive than a specific (individual) face. In addition to studies conducted on samples from America or Europe (Perrett, 2010), research has been conducted on other groups, ethnicities, or cultures – evidence has been found, for example, in China and Japan (Rhodes et al., 2001), among the Hadza tribe in Tanzania (Apicella et al., 2007), and in South Africa (Coetzee et al., 2014). The beauty of averageness is thus based on two principles – the evolutionary tendency to prefer individuals without deviations and peculiarities, and the process of creating a prototype of a beautiful face based on experience (Démuthová, 2023).

Sexually dimorphic traits are a visible reflection of sexual differentiation predominantly associated with hormone levels. These traits are significantly related to the reproductive capacity of an organism, which is a crucial characteristic in an evolutionary context. Studies analyzing beautiful female faces have found that typically feminine features include higher arched eyebrows, a narrower nasal bridge, smaller jaw, fuller lips with a more pronounced philtrum and "Cupid's bow", and a smaller lower face (Little et al., 2011A; Bannister et al., 2022). The presence of feminine facial features not only enhances the overall attractiveness of a woman's face (Little et al., 2014; Foo et al., 2017; Bannister et al., 2022) but also indicates her health and fertility (see, e.g., Little et al., 2011a; Gray & Boothroyd, 2012; Little et al., 2014; Zelazniewicz et al., 2021). L. S. Pflüger et al. even found that the association of facial femininity with fertility is evident not only in potential fertility (i.e., better chances of conceiving, carrying, and delivering offspring) but also in actual fertility – women who exhibited higher levels of feminine facial features in their youth had more offspring than women with less pronounced signs of femininity (Pflüger et al., 2012). On the other hand, a beautiful male face is characterized, in the context of sexually dimorphic traits, by a massive jaw, prominent cheekbones with less subcutaneous fat and tissue (Little et al., 2011a), a generally wide face with a large and massive lower part, thin lips, a wide interorbital distance, and a broad nose (Mitteroecker et al., 2015). Research has demonstrated, for example, the correlation between masculine facial features and sperm quality in men

(Foo et al., 2017), as well as with a wide range of health indicators in adolescent boys (Rhodes et al., 2003).

Another example of features that significantly enhance the beauty of the human face (though this potential list of influential characteristics certainly is not exhaustive) is neoteny. Features of a youthful (not childlike) face indicate that an individual is not too old for reproduction (preservation and spread of genes). Aging brings about changes that are not favorable from an evolutionary perspective (the law of entropy – Gilbert, 2000) – with aging comes the accumulation of a wide range of molecular and cellular damages, a decrease in physical and mental capacity, an increasing risk of diseases, and ultimately death (World Health Organization: WHO, 2022), along with the deterioration of functions necessary for survival and fertility (Gilbert, 2000). An older organism – compared to a younger one – is more likely to exhibit dysfunctions and diseases as well as a lower expected remaining lifespan. Aging is accompanied by the accumulation of damages to macromolecules such as DNA, RNA, proteins, and lipids (Maynard et al., 2015), and it is notable that the ability of the organism to repair these damages significantly declines with age (Gorbunova et al., 2007). This means that younger individuals are generally not only healthier, more resilient, and more vigorous than older ones but also have a higher likelihood that their genetic material, which they transmit to their offspring, will be of higher quality. Studies have shown that youthful facial features significantly enhance the evaluation of beauty especially in women (Kuraguchi et al., 2015; Zheng et al., 2018); however, they also have their significance in the evaluation of male facial beauty (Doi et al., 2017).

With a certain level of generalization, it can be stated that a beautiful human face belongs to a healthy organism capable not only of survival but also of ensuring survival for its future generations. However, how is it possible to identify evolutionary principles for the beauty of non-human and inanimate objects? Evolution relies not only on the principles of sexual selection, which have been dominant interpretive frameworks in explaining the features of beautiful figures and faces, but also on the principles of natural selection, which are much broader. It is through these principles that features influencing the evaluation of their beauty can also be identified in inanimate objects.

Beautiful Objects

The evolutionary significance of traits associated with beauty, such as indicators of good health, genes, or developmental stability, would be challenging to discern in inanimate objects. However, characteristics such as symmetry or averageness demonstrate that many features of beautiful individuals are also present in non-human objects. Practically, this is evidenced by the preference of certain artistic works by a broad segment of the population, the massive attendance at particular sites, or natural sceneries, and so forth. The (almost) universal preference for objects that contain or are distinguished by certain characteristics (e.g., symmetry, averageness) to a greater extent than other objects is reflected in the fact that we find them more appealing. The evolutionary basis of this tendency can be observed in the advantages such objects offer for survival. In the case of symmetry, these include effectiveness, comprehensibility, and predictability.

Effectiveness refers to the amount of energy required for the perceptual and cognitive processing of an object. Nature inherently employs methods and solutions that are the most energy-efficient, meaning the expenditure of the least amount of energy with the greatest benefit. Perceiving complex and intricate objects demands considerable time and attention, which is a significant disadvantage – in a competitive and hazardous environment involving the struggle for survival, resources, or mates, the need to focus intensely and expend substantial energy on observing and analyzing an object is a burden and a considerable drawback. From this perspective, symmetrical objects are optimal for perceptual efficiency, and the cognitive apparatus demonstrably prefers them (Little, 2014). For example, with symmetry along one axis, only half the time is needed to capture the entire object; with two axes, it is only a quarter of the time, and so forth. Additionally, when the cognitive apparatus analyses part of an object, the other part (in the case of symmetry along one axis) is already known, which further enhances the object's beauty – familiar things evoke a sense of safety and positive reactions, and thus are rated as more beautiful.

This aspect is even more pronounced in the context of another facet of symmetrical or average objects, comprehensibility. The primary function of perception is to acquire information, and information is useful only if it can be understood and if critical details can be abstracted. Unintelligible data are a burden; an individual spends excessive time processing them, and their utility remains questionable. Processing complex and ambiguous information/objects requires significantly more energy and attention from the cognitive apparatus (Mudrik et al., 2011), necessitates longer processing times, and yields less accurate results (Davenport & Potter, 2004; Underwood, 2005). Symmetrical objects generally have the ability to clearly communicate the underlying principle on which they are based. The rapid and straightforward detection of the rules governing an object's construction enables not only swift (and thus efficient) perception (Démuth et al., 2019) but also provides the perceiver with additional critical information – it conveys the principles of the object's construction and arrangement, ultimately making it comprehensible. The importance and preference for comprehensible objects in terms of perception have been confirmed by various studies – meaningful stimuli dominate over abstract ones (Yu & Blake, 1992); well-organized structures are highly preferred in visual processing (Mühlenbeck et al., 2016). Conversely, the identification of unintelligible or incongruent objects is significantly hindered. Symmetry, as a principle, greatly facilitates the comprehensibility of objects – the identification of a symmetrical object by the perceiver from different perspectives is much easier than the identification of other patterns (Enquist & Arak, 1994); symmetry also significantly eases the segmentation of the perceived object (Machilsen et al., 2009). The evolutionary preference for symmetry, therefore, stems from the ease with which objects are processed, reinforced by the positive emotions accompanying this perception – the easier (faster, more efficient) the processing of an object, the more intense the aesthetic response (Reber et al., 2004). Similarly, the concept of averageness can be considered – when we perceive an object that closely resembles the prototype of objects we commonly encounter within a particular category; we recognize and understand it much better than an object that is unfamiliar and deviates from what we have previously encountered.

Predictability is the pinnacle of cognition – even science, in its methods of inquiry (description, explanation, and prediction), places the prediction of phenomena at the highest level (Greenwood, 1989). Prediction allows an organism to foresee the consequences of potential events and choose the best alternative (Budaev et al., 2019). In this regard, symmetrical objects are highly predictable both in the short and long term. Short-term predictability reflects the fact that if symmetry is present and we know only part of an object, we can predict how the rest will appear, even with relatively little information. Potentially missing (or not yet perceived) details can thus be easily compensated for by good predictability – symmetry enables a high degree of perceptual fluency (Reber, 2002), and numerous studies have repeatedly confirmed that smooth perceptual processing leads to positive hedonic feelings (Makin et al., 2012; Bertamini & Makin, 2014). Long-term predictability of symmetrical objects is based on the fact that the presence of symmetry signals developmental stability over time. It is therefore expected that symmetrical objects will retain their stability in the future, making it more likely that we can accurately predict their appearance and behavior compared to asymmetrical objects. Averageness also significantly contributes to predictability – due to the higher similarity of a new object to the prototype of previously perceived objects within a given category, it is possible to estimate greater similarity in properties and future behavior. Familiarity and predictability are again rewarded with positive emotions in the form of experiences of beauty and attractiveness (Faerber et al., 2016).

In the context of evolutionarily oriented interpretations of the tendency to attribute aesthetic value to certain features of objects, it can be stated that the pressures of natural and sexual selection have led to the preference for specific characteristics that advantaged individuals in the competitive struggle (for survival or a mate) and increased the likelihood of their genes' survival and success. Since these characteristics are often hidden, a strong tendency toward high sensitivity to their external manifestations has developed. The significant benefits that such detection ability caused likely led to the evolution of the ability of detection and preference for certain characteristics (through their external signs, i.e., signals) in both human and non-human objects into specific brain activity, accompanied by intense and positive emotional responses (experiences of liking, beauty). Evolutionarily conditioned preferences were thus reinforced with each perception of beautiful objects, as these elicited a positive emotional response that rewarded the discovery or preference of a beautiful object over a less attractive one.

Beauty and the Brain

An undeniable testament to the significance of perceiving beautiful objects in the phylogeny of humans is the formation of unique neural connections that are specifically active in the brain during aesthetic experiences. Neuroaesthetic models of perception and processing of information about beautiful objects have been refined with the accumulation of research findings and the improvement of available (particularly imaging) techniques. Early models by Zeki, Ramachandran, and Hirstein posited that "visual objects are discriminated by peak shift effect; then, features are extracted and grouped into unitary clusters by different visual areas; a certain feature which is special importance is reinforced by activation of both limbic structures and allocation of attentional resources to produce pleasurable rewarding sensations" (Li & Zhang, 2020, p. 4). Subsequently, Anjan Chatterjee (Chatterjee & Vartanian, 2014) specified that three main neural systems are involved in the process of aesthetic experience: the sensory-motor system, the emotion-valuation system, and the knowledge-meaning system. This highlighted the broad range of processes that the perception and evaluation of beautiful objects encompass. In the context of the variety of mechanisms involved in the perception and evaluation of beauty, Redies pointed out that aesthetic perception comprises two distinct processes: "aesthetics of perception" and "aesthetics of cognition" (Redies, 2015). According to Redies, "perceptual processing is based on the intrinsic form of an artwork, which may or may not be beautiful. If it is beautiful, a beauty-responsive mechanism is activated in the brain. This bottom-up mechanism is universal amongst humans; it is widespread in the visual brain and responsive across visual modalities... The cognitive processing is based on contextual information, such as the depicted content, the intentions of the artist, or the circumstances of the presentation of the artwork. Cognitive processing is partially top-down and varies between individuals according to their cultural experience. Processing in the two channels is parallel and largely independent. In the general case, an aesthetic experience is induced if processing in both channels is favorable, i.e., if there is resonance in the perceptual processing channel ('aesthetics of perception'), and successful mastering in the cognitive processing channel ('aesthetics of cognition')" (Redies, 2015, 1). He also speculated, that this combinatorial mechanism has evolved to mediate social bonding between members of a (cultural) group of people. Also, what is important, primary emotions can be elicited via both channels and modulate the degree of the aesthetic experience.

A crucial piece of information related to brain activity during aesthetic tasks is the activation of the reward circuit – brain regions innervated by dopamine pathways (Liang et al., 2010). These include primarily the nucleus accumbens and the orbitofrontal cortex (Cloutier et al., 2008). Importantly, this activation is associated with positive emotions, which function as a reward and reinforce behavior that leads to the elicitation of these positive emotions. This reinforcement results in a desire to repeatedly expose oneself to beautiful objects and to continually experience these positive feelings.

It is therefore evident that the search for and preference for beautiful objects has its evolutionary justification. Evolutionary contexts of investigating the issue of beauty are, of course, only one of many factors and explanatory levels that offer their own perspective on beauty. Like other approaches, evolutionary theories emphasize a certain type of influence (biological) and do not focus on other factors (cultural, psychological, etc.). They have their own methods and procedures, but precisely because of their focus, they allow the revelation of aspects of beauty from their specific viewpoint, which can contribute to a comprehensive understanding of this multifaceted and complex issue.

Linguistic Contexts

In addition to philosophical, historical, biological, and psychological approaches to studying beauty, the analysis of its usage in natural language is an important source of information for understanding the concept. Language reflects not only cultural context but also historical experiences that integrate the knowledge of the language users. Working with language offers numerous approaches represented by diverse techniques of analyzing language and the concept of beauty, each with the potential to capture and reflect different types of information. Etymology, along with content analysis of historical texts on beauty, allows for the tracing of the development and understanding of the concept back to its roots – identifying overlaps with related languages, searching for potential sources of semantic deviations formed during its evolution, as well as the extensive contexts in which the term "beauty" appears in historical texts. Content and frequency analyses of the connotations of the term "beauty" provide information that beauty is very often associated with individuals who are not only sources of positive aesthetic experiences but also significant objects for an individual, appreciated for representing important values. In this context, it is interesting to observe how certain patterns of thought associated with the perception of beauty (e.g., beauty as a value) appear across historical periods and how they also chronically emerge as salient features identified through completely different methodological approaches applied today.

Etymology

Examining the terms used in different languages to denote beauty reveals that the basic terms for this concept often stem from entirely different etymological roots. For instance, M. M. Rakhmatova analyzed the original meanings of beauty in English, Uzbek, and Tajik. In the etymological dictionary of the Uzbek language, the word "beautiful" means a connection with a beautiful face, and in Old Turkic, it essentially means appearance. In the Tajik language, the word "zeboi" etymologically refers to the term "oroish", which means to adorn oneself (Rakhmatova, 2019). According to the etymological English dictionary, the term "beauty" is linked to the word "bealte" from the 14th century, denoting physical attractiveness but also goodness and courtesy (Etymonline, 2023). At this level, it can already be observed that beauty can be associated with diverse concepts pointing to both aesthetic (face, appearance) and axiomatic (goodness) levels of understanding. *Etymonline* further states that the term beauty comes from the earlier Anglo-French term "beute", Old French (12th century) "biauté" (modern French "beauté") with meanings: beauty, seductiveness, beautiful person. An even earlier term is "beletet" from Vulgar Latin, derived from "bellitatem" (in the nominative form: "bellitas") expressing "a state of pleasure to the senses" (Etymonline, 2023). *The Cambridge Advanced Learner's Dictionary* describes beauty as "a quality that gives pleasure, especially by being looked at, or someone or something that gives great pleasure, especially when looked at" (McIntosh, 2013, p. 125). The primary meaning of the English term is therefore associated with a pleasant sensory stimulus. On the other hand, the *Oxford Advanced Learner's Dictionary* extends the definition by defining beauty as "a quality that pleases the senses or the mind" (Hornby, 2011, p. 119).

Beauty does not have to be linked solely to sensory qualities (it does not reside only in the eye, ear, etc., of the beholder), but it is also an object of rational or mental pleasure. Similar sensory "logic" of beauty can be found in Turkish, German, or Swedish. According to Nisanyan (2011), the Turkish word for beauty ("güzel") originates from Old Turkish and evolved from the word "gözel", which in Middle Turkish means pleasant form – beautiful. In Swedish, beauty derives from the Old Germanic "vacker" ("wakraz"), which refers to a pleasant, sweet taste. The Hebrew "hpy" ("Yapheh") expresses appropriateness, regularity, and order, which are attributes related more to cognitive than sensory qualities. It seems that different cultures/environments valued and appreciated different qualities as beautiful. These influences can be considered a continuation of the evolutionary pressures that, in the early phases of human phylogeny, caused certain objects to be considered beautiful because they indicated other (evolutionarily advantageous) qualities of the organism.

A. Démuth et al. analyzed the etymological roots of the concept of beauty in Slavic, Germanic, Semitic, and Romance languages, as well as in Turkish (Démuth et al., 2023). Similar to the origin of the English word "beauty", which primarily refers to the visual qualities of an object, the German term "die Schönheit" (Swedish "skönhet") refers to visibility (in Old High German: Scōni "ansehnlich" – Pfeifer et al., 1993) and appearance ("schauen"). The root of this word thus indicates that beauty is related not only to the ability to see but also to pay attention, observe, and look. Greek has several terms denoting beauty, the most basic being "κάλλος". "Kallos" primarily denotes the beauty of the body (Liddell & Scott, 1940), secondarily the beauty of an individual – initially mostly men, then other objects as well. R. J. Cunliffe in *"A Lexicon of the Homeric Dialect"* states that the primary meaning of the term "kallos" is indeed the beauty of a man (Cunliffe, 1924), and only subsequently can this term be used to denote things such as clothing and jewelry, items that embellish the bearer (Liddell & Scott, 1940). A similar ontologizing understanding of beauty can be found in some Slavic languages. In Russian, for example, the term for beauty uses words derived from the Old Slavic designation of the red color (краса / красота/ *krasьnъ – Derksen, 2008). The Proto-Slavic "krasa" was associated with shine, redness, the color of fire, and the Proto-Slavic "kresati" (Rejzek, 2001). The concise etymological dictionary of Slovak states its connection with fire, but primarily with adornment, embellishment, and decoration (Králik, 2015).

It is evident that the roots of the concept of beauty indicate the nuances and variations in its meanings, as well as the multidimensionality of this concept. This multidimensionality can be perceived, for instance, through intersections with other words that are considered synonyms or related terms to beauty. The following paragraphs, therefore, focus on identifying the similarities (as well as differences) between the concept of beauty and related terms. Analyses aimed at identifying the connotations of the term "beauty", similarities in the semantic differentials of beauty and related terms, and text analyses centered on the concept of beauty confirm that the study of language and its usage by ordinary users represents a significant source of information.

Related Concepts

There are several ways to investigate what the concept of beauty signifies in language. Beyond analyzing extensive texts (for instance, through the method of latent semantic analysis, which uses statistical computations applied to a collection of documents to extract meaning from texts such as sentences, paragraphs, or essays), it is possible to elicit expressions from language users that they associate with the target concept (so-called connotations) or to examine the relatedness of terms using the semantic differential method, which measures the extent and in which areas (adjectives) two terms are closely related. Another valuable source of information can be synonym dictionaries, which characterize the concept of beauty through related terms within a given language. In Slovak, for example, the term "krása" (beauty) is associated with: beauty – an attribute of what is nice, beautiful: beauty (feminine beauty), splendor (splendor of nature), magnificence (magnificence of a temple), picturesqueness (picturesqueness of a landscape), gracefulness (gracefulness of shapes), charm (the charm of village houses), attractiveness, and breathtakingness (the breathtakingness of a picture) (Synonymický slovník slovenčiny, 2004).

Another approach is research focused on identifying the connotations of the concept of beauty among ordinary language users. For instance, studies with Slovak participants have shown (detailed results can be found in Démuthová & Démuth, 2021) that the most frequent connotations of the term "beauty" are nature (this connotation appeared in 35.28% of the surveyed sample), woman (21.73%), love (17.77%), family (15.02%), child (15.02%), and flower (10.93%). It is evident that beauty relates to people (woman, child), surrounding objects (nature, flower), as well as to values (love, family). In literature, however, there is a very frequent association between beauty and goodness. This connection stems from various sources – ranging from etymology ("bealte" = physical attractiveness, goodness, and courtesy – Harper, 2023), through evolutionary perspectives (beauty as a signal of quality), to philosophical concepts (the ancient concept of kalokagathia – Eco, 2005), and it also appears in language (e.g., a well-crafted and artistically mastered painting might be described as "beautifully painted," even if it does not appeal to us aesthetically, but rather conveys that it is well executed). Despite the frequent association and occasional interchangeability between beauty and goodness, the concept of goodness ranked only 19th among connotations in the mentioned study, with a 3.7% representation (Démuthová & Démuth, 2021).

Other analytical methods, however, indicate that beauty and goodness are indeed concepts that are closely related (detailed results are available in Démuthová & Démuth, 2023a). Using the semantic differential method (Osgood, 1957; Osgood et al., 1957) – a procedure that allows for the measurement of subjective evaluations of a specific term through a series of bipolar adjective pairs (see Table 1) – the characteristics of the concepts of beauty and goodness were examined. In a semantic differential, an individual evaluates a selected term (in our case beauty) on a scale (typically seven-point) based on how close or far the term is to one of two opposing adjectives (e.g., pleasant/unpleasant, fast/slow, etc.). Based on this evaluation, the term is assigned a value on a specific scale (e.g., a scale of pleasantness or speed), which can then be represented in the space between two points corresponding to the two opposing adjectives. The advantage of this method is that, in addition to providing information about the nature of the relationship between two concepts (the evaluated term and the adjective), the result is quantifiable (indicating how close the term is to the adjective), and the clear, resultant evaluations can be used for comparison with other terms. Since the semantic differential provides data in a quantitative form, it is possible to conduct meta-analysis through factor analysis. Osgood et al. (1957) identified three basic

Table 1. Bipolar adjectives used to describe the concepts of Beauty and Goodness and their categorization into the dimensions of activity, evaluation, and potency

Dimensions	Activity	Evaluation	Potency
Bipolar Adjectives	Exciting/Soothing	Inviting/Repulsive	Orderly/Chaotic
	Aggressive/Moderate	Inspiring/Boring	Balanced/Unbalanced
	Erotic/Romantic	Kind/Hateful	Understandable/Unintelligible
	Expressive/Inconspicuous	Calm/Restless	Logical/Illogical
	Strict/Lenient	Pure/Dirty	Knowable/Unknowable
	Impulsive/Judicious	Pleasant/Unpleasant	Familiar/Strange
	Fast/Slow	Good/Bad	Simple/Complicated

Source: Démuthová & Démuth (2023a, 4)

universal dimensions: strength (potency), activity, and evaluation, which have been demonstrated across a wide range of studies and which we also used for researching the relatedness of the concepts of beauty and goodness (see Table 1).

The results of the comparison of semantic differentials for the words "beauty" and "goodness" indicate that out of the twenty-one bipolar adjectives used to evaluate the concepts of beauty and goodness, a difference was identified in only three (Démuthová & Démuth, 2023a) – beauty is more exciting, impulsive, and illogical compared to goodness. These differences can be attributed to the nature of the concepts under investigation – while beauty is primarily associated with aesthetic evaluation, goodness is related to morality. Aesthetic evaluations are characterized by their intensity and immediacy, which explains the association with excitement and impulsivity (Schindler et al., 2017). On the other hand, moral evaluations also involve evaluative aspects (Tangney et al., 2007) and engage considerations (closely associated with the adjective "logical"), which may be less pronounced in aesthetic evaluations. The overall similarity between the concepts of beauty and goodness, as demonstrated in the analysis of semantic differentials, aligns with the tendencies evident in well-known stereotypes (e.g., the "what is beautiful is good stereotype" – Dion et al., 1972) and cognitive biases (e.g., the "halo effect" – Nisbett & Wilson, 1977) described primarily in social psychology. It is thus evident that not only language but also these stereotypes and biases contribute to the shared characteristics exhibited by the concepts of beauty and goodness.

Slightly different results obtained from comparing the semantic differentials of the concepts of beauty and goodness (demonstrating the closeness of the concepts) and the results of the analysis of the connotations of the term "beauty" (where the term "goodness" ranked only 19th) also highlight the significant importance of the methodology used in scientific inquiry. It has long been recognized that the perspective, chosen approach, and method of investigation significantly influence the results obtained. The method (from the Greek methodos = path to a goal – Králik, 2015) serves as both the path and the decisive means to knowledge. However, the chosen path of approaching a problem also directly influences the conclusions we reach about the object under study. Therefore, the method to a certain (and often considerable) extent predetermines what we learn about the subject of study. The exploration of beauty serves as an exemplary case of a problem addressed by numerous scientific disciplines such as aesthetics (Dietrich & Knieper, 2022), art (Sidhu et al., 2018), psychology (Yarosh, 2019), medicine (Feng, 2020), mathematics (Zeki et al., 2018), philosophy (Scruton, 2011), and biology (Jones & Jaeger, 2019). Each of these disciplines employs its own methods of investigation, analyzes different aspects of beauty, uses specific terminology, and perceives the importance of different outcomes. Another platform that intensively explores the relationship between beauty and goodness is neuroaesthetics. Through various techniques for mapping brain activity, it has been shown, for example, that aesthetic and moral judgments share the same brain activity. Research by Tsukiura and Cabeza (2011) demonstrated that activity in the medial orbitofrontal cortex increased as a function of both attractiveness and goodness ratings. Additionally, within each of these regions, "the activations elicited by attractiveness and goodness judgments were strongly correlated with each other, supporting the idea of similar contributions of each region to both judgments" (Tsukiura & Cabeza, 2011, p. 138). Once again, the thesis "what is beautiful is good" is confirmed, this time at the neural level.

Opposites

In addition to identifying related concepts and expressions, it is also important to analyze the mutual relationship between the concept of beauty and its opposites. Certain characteristics of objects and phenomena become visible only when contrasted with the characteristics of different or contrary terms. One of the concepts most frequently examined as an opposite to beauty is ugliness (see, for example, Dietrich & Knieper, 2022; Martin-Loeches et al., 2014). The Thesaurus for the English Language lists the strongest opposites of the concept of beauty as: crudeness, inelegance, and roughness (Thesaurus, 2024). Ugliness is also often cited as a prominent opposite to beauty (see e.g., Lan et al., 2021). On the other hand, several authors point out that ugliness and beauty can coexist in some domains (Felisberti, 2022) – examples of this can be observed in the concept of wabi-sabi (Garcia, 2015), the appreciation of ugliness in art (Eco, 2007), or even in architecture (e.g., brutalism –Sibbald, 2016).

Similarly to the examination of the mutual proximity of the concepts of beauty and goodness, an analysis comparing the semantic differentials of the concepts of beauty and ugliness was conducted. The same set of bipolar adjectives was used for evaluating the concepts (see Table 1). From the results (for detailed insights see Démuthová & Démuth, 2023b), it is apparent that although beauty and ugliness are antonyms, this does not automatically imply that they have opposite meanings at all levels. Statistically significant differences were not shown in one pair out of the twenty-one bipolar adjectives: "impulsive/judicious". Thus, the term "ugliness" appears to be a relatively apt opposite to the concept of beauty. From the results of the comparison of semantic differentials, it is also possible to determine which characteristics are most typical for the concept of beauty, and conversely, which ones (in the context of comparing beauty and ugliness) depict the concept of ugliness. For beauty, these included pleasant, inviting, and inspiring, while ugliness was characterized as unpleasant, repulsive, and bad. In addition to specific findings in the form of results indicating differences between the concepts of beauty and ugliness, it is important to note that the chosen methodology (semantic differential, especially with a representative selection of twenty-one bipolar adjectives) effectively differentiated between the assessed concepts. This means that there is a procedure available that can be utilized in further research and for evaluating other concepts.

From the examples provided, it is evident that the study of language can be a highly beneficial domain for investigating the concept of beauty and its meanings. It is also clear that most approaches are yet to fully utilize their potential in the field of studying beauty in language – we have effective and sensitive methods, and the development of computer programs capable of analyzing extensive corpora and tracking multifaceted relationships between concepts is advancing the research possibilities of the meaning of beauty into unexplored realms. The complexity, multidimensionality, and, last but not least, the inherent attractiveness of beauty as an object of scientific inquiry open up broad and appealing opportunities for further exploration by researchers.

Specific Contexts

From the analyses of comparisons of semantic differentials of the concept of beauty and related or distinct concepts, it is evident that interpreting the results requires considering several intervening variables. The data described above suggest that the understanding of the concept of beauty may be influenced by language itself, as well as various cultural (Jacobsen, 2010) or temporal (Sorokowski, 2010) specifics. Studies focusing on factors that can modify the concept of beauty in individuals and groups further demonstrate that the understanding of this concept may also depend on age (Wulff et al., 2022), motivational aspects (Mirfazeli et al., 2021), or even hormonal changes over the course of life and relatively short periods of time (Marcinkowska et al., 2018).

In this context (as an example of how and to what extent/in what areas individual factors can modify the understanding of the concept of beauty), we present the results of research conducted on the Slovak population, examining the effect of gender, age, and education on the understanding of the concept of beauty. These examples highlight how individual variables can enter into the understanding of beauty – for example, gender, as a variable that is rarely considered when defining and delineating concepts, showed a greater effect on the understanding of the concept of beauty than artistic education, which is perceived more as a path leading to diametrically different perspectives and evaluations of what we consider beautiful. Results contradicting the established mindset indicate that empirical research in the areas of beauty studies is necessary and brings interesting and novel insights.

Age

The content of the concept of beauty is the subject of ongoing research – these studies (as we have already indicated) bring interesting insights, but at the same time, they highlight the need to consider several intervening variables in analyses and interpretations that may modify the understanding of this term. One of several variables whose influence on the concept of beauty is considered is age. Studies focusing on this factor are rare (see, e.g., Salehi et al., 2019; He et al., 2021). Some studies show a tendency for older participants to rate facial beauty more leniently – younger participants are more critical in evaluating facial attractiveness (see, e.g., Ebner et al., 2018; Kiiski et al., 2016). There are several studies examining the effect of experience on the assessment of beauty – for example, Ardizzi et al. (2023) found that sensorimotor experience with a certain quality of an object leads to objects possessing that quality being perceived as more beautiful. What is known, frequent, familiar,... is considered more beautiful (Démuthová et al., 2019). Experience as such can thus be an important factor in the perception and evaluation of beauty.

Based on these facts, it can be assumed that there might be differences in the understanding of the concept of beauty between younger and older participants. To verify this, we used a validated method of semantic differential as well as a method of analyzing the most frequent connotations of the concept of beauty depending on the age of respondents in a Slovak sample of participants (see Démuthová & Démuth, 2024a; 2024b). In the semantic differential method, the same set of bipolar adjectives was used (see Table 1), and the statistical analysis of the assessment of the proximity of these adjectives to the concept of beauty showed that most (eleven) bipolar adjectives characterizing the concept of beauty (especially in the dimension of potency) correlate statistically significantly with age. With increasing age, the concept of beauty is characterized as more simple, understandable, logical, knowable, orderly, balanced, less impulsive, exciting, and inspiring. Interpretations of the results suggest a tendency toward gradual calming and greater stability of individuals in older age, as well as the possibility of better self-awareness or identification (based on a greater volume of experience) of key characteristics of what characterizes beautiful objects (Démuthová & Démuth, 2024a). Analysis of the most frequent connotations of the concept of beauty in relation to age (Démuthova & Démuth, 2024b) showed relative stability in the content of the concept of beauty over time. It thus seems that the content of this concept remains relatively stable throughout life; what changes is the dynamics with which individuals approach the perception of the concept of beauty.

Gender

When considering how the understanding of the concept of beauty changes depending on gender, research studies are mostly cited reflecting the differences in preferences based on whether we evaluate the beauty of men or the beauty of women. A beautiful woman (as partially indicated in the previous subchapter "Beautiful Body") is in her fertile age (Bovet et al., 2018), has a body indicating the ability to conceive and bear a child (Singh, 2002), healthy skin (Jones et al., 2004), and a symmetrical face (Scheib et al., 1999). A handsome man has broad shoulders, is tall (Pazhoohi et al., 2023), strong (Sell et al., 2017), and dominant (Rahal et al., 2021). Research in this area is rich and suggests many evolutionary or socially conditioned preferences in assessing the beauty of others, especially in the context of interpersonal interactions.

A less explored area is how men and women perceive beauty in general – as a complex that encompasses its various forms. In this regard, research has been conducted focusing on differences in the connotations of the concept of beauty between genders (Vavrová & Démuthová, 2021), as well as in the semantic differential of the concept of beauty (Démuthová & Démuth, 2023c). In the context of monitoring, the most frequent connotations of the concept of beauty at the top two positions for men were connotations that refer to persons of the opposite sex in the interpersonal proximity of the man ("wife" and "girlfriend"). Further down in the order of significance were more abstract connotations ("beauty" and "aesthetics"), followed again by more concrete terms like "figure" and "woman". Adjectives "beautiful" and "inner" ranked seventh and ninth, respectively, while words like "nature" and "love" also made it into the top ten typical connotations of the concept of beauty produced by men. All ten of the most significant connotations for men were of the feminine gender (including adjectives "beautiful" and "inner"), indicating the mentioned close association with ideas of the opposite sex (Vavrová & Démuthová, 2021).

The list of the ten most preferred connotations of the concept of beauty for women is similar in many respects to the list for men – new entries include connotations such as "grandchild" (in 4th place), "youth" (6th place), "God", and "happiness" (9th and 10th place). Interestingly, women also placed connotations "wife" and "woman" in prominent positions, rather than their male counterparts (which would be "husband" and "man"). Among the typical connotations for female participants were also nouns like "nature", "aesthetics", "beauty", and the sole adjective "beautiful". The results indicate a strong connection in women between the meaning of the concept of beauty and family (evidenced by expressions like: "wife", "woman", "grandchild"), as well as with the role of women as mothers (and grandmothers). However, this role is contingent on a woman's fertility, which (unlike that of a man) diminishes during active life and is therefore associated with youth (the term "youth" ranked 6th). Family ties and their continuity are thus a source of pleasure for women to such an extent that they are directly associated with deep aesthetic experiences (Vavrová & Démuthová, 2021).

Education

Examining the effect of education on the understanding of the concept of beauty stems from the assumption that academic environments have a significant liberalizing influence (Dey, 1996) and are characterized by cognitive sophistication (Gelepithis & Giani, 2022). These, in turn, lead to more open attitudes and opinions; for example, it has been shown that with increasing levels of education, the occurrence of prejudices (Kuppens & Spears, 2014; Scott, 2022) and negative attitudes significantly decreases (Rivera-Garrido, 2022). It can therefore be assumed that the understanding of the concept of Beauty among more educated individuals will be more complex; they will be more open-minded and less conservative in their evaluations.

The understanding of the concept of beauty may be influenced not only by academic education but also by artistic education. Artists encounter beautiful objects, subject them to closer scrutiny, and gradually develop a greater ability to perceive Beauty (Cantekin Elyağutu, 2016). They are also trained to find aspects of beauty in unconventional or unusual situations and contexts. Creative and artistic education, for example, leads to a greater openness to new experiences (Ulger, 2016) and respect for the artistic traditions of various nations (Vladimirova et al., 2019). Due to training in openness and the ability to find Beauty in various forms, it is assumed that individuals with artistic education will have a broader view of the definition of Beauty. Moreover, compared to individuals without an artistic background, they may be more active in this area.

These assumptions were empirically tested using the semantic differential method – it was found that differences in the understanding of the concept of Beauty between people with artistic education and laypeople, and between individuals with higher and lower levels of academic education, are rare (for detailed results, see Démuthová & Démuth, 2024). Out of twenty-one bipolar adjectives, individuals with higher academic education differed from those with lower academic education in only two: individuals with higher education perceived beauty as slower and more lenient than those with lower education. It is possible that a higher level of academic education teaches individuals to be more thoughtful, and to avoid hasty or impulsive conclusions. The development of critical thinking in college students is one of the desired outcomes of higher education (Bellaera et al., 2021). Therefore, when encountering Beauty, individuals with higher levels of education may tend to explore, analyze, and avoid making hasty conclusions. Critical thinking strengthened by education is also associated with curiosity, flexibility in evaluating stereotypes or prejudices, openness to differences and possibilities, caution in decision-making, and willingness to consider and revise one's position through reflection (Yuan et al., 2020). These are all characteristics that generally lead to leniency rather than strict judgments. Differences were found in the evaluation of beauty between individuals without artistic education and those with artistic education in three out of twenty-one bipolar adjectives – once again, it can be concluded that artistic education, although appearing as a significant variable, has only a small impact on how laypeople and artists perceive beauty.

Conclusion

Beauty is a multidimensional and multidisciplinary concept. In its examination, it is essential to consider the perspectives of each of the involved scientific disciplines along with their specific research methodologies. Besides scientific inquiry, it is beneficial to observe how the concept of beauty is handled by the general language user (layperson) and to take into account the historical, cultural, and geographical specifics that influence the meaning of this concept. Beauty encompasses both objective and subjective aspects – its perception is, in many respects, based on evolutionarily conditioned mechanisms, while its specific manifestations are significantly influenced by contemporary trends and individual taste. The considerable diversity of forms in which beauty is presented offers a wide range of areas for study; however, due to its variability, it defies clear definition. It is perhaps for this reason that beauty has inspired humanity for millennia and continues to be a challenge.

References

Agnew, P., & Koella, J. C. (1997). Virulence, parasite mode of transmission, and host fluctuating asymmetry. *Proceedings. Biological Sciences, 264*(1378), 9–15. https://doi.org/10.1098/rspb.1997.0002

Apicella, C. L., Little, A. C., & Marlowe, F. W. (2007). Facial averageness and attractiveness in an isolated population of hunter-gatherers. *Perception, 36*(12), 1813–1820. https://doi.org/10.1068/p5601

Ardizzi, M., Ferroni, F., Manini, A., Giudici, C., Maccaferri, E., Uccelli, S., & Umiltà, M. A. (2023). The influence of sensorimotor experience on beauty evaluation of preschool children. *Frontiers in Human Neuroscience, 17*, 1138420. https://doi.org/10.3389/fnhum.2023.1138420

Aristotle. (2004). *The Metaphisics*. Penguin Books

Bannister, J. J., Juszczak, H., Aponte, J. D., Katz, D. C., Knott, P. D., Weinberg, S. M., Hallgrímsson, B., Forkert, N. D., & Seth, R. (2022). Sex differences in adult facial three-dimensional morphology: application to gender-affirming facial surgery. *Facial Plastic Surgery & Aesthetic Medicine, 24*(2), 24–30. https://doi.org/10.1089/fpsam.2021.0301

Bascom, J. (1867). *Aesthetics; or, the Science of Beauty*. Crosby and Ainsworth.

Bellaera, L., Weinstein-Jones, Y., Ilie, S., & Baker, S.T. (2021). Critical thinking in practice: the priorities and practices of instructors teaching in higher education. *Thinking Skills and Creativity, 41*(4), 100856. https://doi.org/10.1016/j.tsc.2021.100856

Bertamini, M., & Makin, A. D. J. (2014). Brain activity in response to visual symmetry. *Symmetry, 6*(4), 975–996. https://doi.org/10.3390/sym6040975

Boëthius, A. M. T. S. (1929). *O útěše filosofie*. [On the Consolation of Philosophy]. Cyrillo-Methodějská kníhtiskárna a nakladatelství V. Kotrba.

Bovet, J., Barkat-Defradas, M., Durand, V., Faurie, C., & Raymond, M. (2018). Women's attractiveness is linked to expected age at menopause. *Journal of Evolutionary Biology, 31*(2), 229–238. https://doi.org/10.1111/jeb.13214

Bowie, A. (2003). *Aesthetics and Subjectivity: From Kant to Nietzsche*. Second edition. Manchester University Press.

Budaev, S., Jørgensen, C., Mangel, M., Eliassen, S., & Giske, J. (2019). Decision-making from the animal perspective: bridging ecology and subjective cognition. *Frontiers in Ecology and Evolution, 7*(1), 164. https://doi.org/10.3389/fevo.2019.00164

Cantekin Elyağutu, D. (2016). Importance of art education. *Art-Sanat, 6*, 243–247. https://dergipark.org.tr/tr/download/article-file/229873

Cao, H. H., Han, B., Hirshleifer, D., & Zhang, H. H. (2011). Fear of the unknown: familiarity and economic decisions. *Review of Finance, 15*(1), 173–206. https://doi.org/10.1093/rof/rfp023

Carleton, N. R. (2016). Fear of the unknown: one fear to rule them all? *Journal of Anxiety Disorders, 41*(1), 5–21. https://doi.org/10.1016/j.janxdis.2016.03.011

Chatterjee, A. & Vartanian, O. (2014). Neuroaesthetics. *Trends in Cognitive Science, 18*(7), 370–375. https://doi.org/10.1016/j.tics.2014.03.003

Cicero, M. T. (1971). *Tusculan Disputations*. Harvard University Press.

Cloutier, J., Heatherton, T. F., Whalen, P. J., & Kelley, W. M. (2008). Are attractive people rewarding? Sex differences in the neural substrates of facial attractiveness. *Journal of Cognitive Neuroscience, 20*(6), 941–951. https://doi.org/10.1162/jocn.2008.20062

Coburn, A., Vartanian, O., & Chatterjee, A. (2017). Buildings, beauty, and the brain: a neuroscience of architectural experience. *Journal of Cognitive Neuroscience, 29*(9), 1521–1531. https://doi.org/10.1162/jocn_a_01146

Coetzee, V., Greeff, J. M., Stephen, I. D., & Perrett, D. I. (2014). Cross-cultural agreement in facial attractiveness preferences: the role of ethnicity and gender. *Plos One, 9*(7), e99629. https://doi.org/10.1371/journal.pone.0099629

Cunliffe, R., J. (1924). *A Lexicon of the Homeric Dialect*. Oxford University Press.

Danescu, A., Rens, E. G., Rehki, J., Woo, J., Akazawa, T., Fu, K., Edelstein-Keshet, L., & Richman, J. M. (2021). Symmetry and fluctuation of cell movements in neural crest-derived facial mesenchyme. *Development, 148*(9). https://doi.org/10.1242/dev.193755

Davenport, J. L., & Potter, M. C. (2004). Scene consistency in object and background perception. *Psychological Science, 15*(8), 559–564. https://doi.org/10.1111/j.0956-7976.2004.00719.x

Démuth, A. (2016). Tri historické matematické prístupy k skúmaniu krásy. [Three Historical Mathematical Approaches to the Study of Beauty]. *Filozofia, 71*(9) 759–770.

Démuth, A. (2019). *Beauty, Aesthetic Experience, and Emotional Affective States*. Peter Lang.

Démuth, A., Démuthová, S., & Keceli, Y. (2023). On some etymological, grammatical and contextual reasons for the vagueness of the concept of beauty. In A. Démuth, & S. Démuthová (eds.), *Conceptual and Semantic Analysis of the Qualitative Domains of Aesthetic and Moral Emotions* (pp. 39-56). Peter Lang.

Démuth, A., & Rušinová, M. (2019). *Cognitive Aesthetics in Classical German Philosophy*. Peter Lang.

Démuthová, S., Démuth, A., & Selecká, L. (2019). *Human Facial Attractiveness in Psychological Research: An Evolutionary Approach*. Peter Lang Verlag.

Démuthová, S. (2023). *Atraktivita ľudskej tváre*. [Attractiveness of the Human Face]. Veda, vydavateľstvo SAV.

Démuthová, S., & Démuth, A. (2021). A frequency and semantic analysis of the most frequent connotations of the notion of beauty. *European Journal of Behavioral Sciences, 4*(1), 1-11. https://doi.org/10.33422/ejbs.v4i1.611

Démuthová, S., & Démuth, A. (2023a). Is beauty good? A comparison of the semantic differentials of the terms beauty and goodness and their gender specificities. In Proceedings of The 7th International Conference on Social Sciences in the 21st Century (1-15). Diamond Scientific Publishing. https://doi.org/10.33422/7th.ics21.2023.09.100

Démuthová, S., & Démuth, A. (2023b). Beauty in the context of ugliness – the similarities and differences of their semantic differentials. In Proceedings of The 7th International Conference on Research in Social Sciences (pp. 13-23). https://doi.org/10.33422/7th.rssconf.2023.07.002

Démuthová, S., & Démuth, A.. (2023c). Semantic differential of the concept of beauty. *Journal of Advanced Research in Social Science, 6*(3), 66-75. https://doi.org/10.33422/jarss.v6i3.1056

Démuthová, S., & Démuth, A. (2024a). How age affects the evaluation of the concept of beauty. In editum.

Démuthová, S., & Démuth, A. (2024b). The relative stability of the concept of beauty across a lifespan. In editum.

Démuthová, S., Kišoňová, R., & Démuth, A. (2024). *Pojem krása. Krása ako estetická emócia.* [The Concept of Beauty: Beauty as an Aesthetic Emotion]. Vydavateľstvo SAV.

Derksen, R. (2007). *Etymological Dictionary of the Slavic Inherited Lexicon*. Brill. Retrieved Feb 22, 2024, from https://brill.com/view/title/12607

Dey, E. L. (1996). Undergraduate political attitudes: an examination of peer, faculty, and social influences. *Research in Higher Education, 37*, 535-554. https://doi.org/10.1007/BF01724937

Dietrich, P., & Knieper, T. (2022). (Neuro)Aesthetics: beauty, ugliness, and ethics. *PsyCh Journal, 11*(5), 619-627. https://doi.org/10.1002/pchj.478

Dion, K. K., Berscheid, E., & Walster, E. (1972). What is beautiful is good. *Journal of Personality and Social Psychology, 24*(3), 285-290. https://doi.org/10.1037/h0033731

Dixson, A. F., Halliwell, G., East, R., Wignarajah, P., & Anderson, M. (2003).

Masculine somatotype and hirsuteness as determinants of sexual attractiveness to women. *Archives of Sexual Behavior, 32*(1), 29–39. https://doi.org/10.1023/a:102188922846

Dixson, B. J., Sagata, K., Linklater, W. L., & Dixson, A. F. (2010). Male preferences for female waist-to-hip ratio and body mass index in the highlands of Papua New Guinea. *American Journal of Physical Anthropology, 141*(4), 620–625. https://doi.org/10.1002/ajpa.21181

Doi, H., Morikawa, M., Inadomi, N., Aikawa, K., Uetani, M., & Shinohara, K. (2017). Neural correlates of babyish adult face processing in men. *Neuropsychologia, 97*, 9–17. https://doi.org/10.1016/j.neuropsychologia.2017.01.017

Dürrigl M. A. (2002). Kalokagathia–beauty is more than just external appearance. *Journal of Cosmetic Dermatology, 1*(4), 208–210. https://doi.org/10.1111/j.1473-2165.2002.00073.x

Ebner, N. C., Luedicke, J., Voelkle, M. C., Riediger, M., Lin, T., & Lindenberger, U. (2018). An adult developmental approach to perceived facial attractiveness and distinctiveness. *Frontiers in Psychology, 9*, 561. https://doi.org/10.3389/fpsyg.2018.00561

Eco U. (2007). *On Ugliness*. Rizzoli.

Eco, U. (2005). *Dějiny krásy*. [On Beauty]. Argo.

Enquist, M., & Arak, A. (1994). Symmetry, beauty and evolution. *Nature, 372*(6502), 169–172. https://doi.org/10.1038/372169a0

Etcoff, N. (1999). *Survival of the Prettiest: The Science of Beauty*. Anchor Books.

Faerber, S. J., Kaufmann, J. M., Leder, H., Martin, E. M., & Schweinberger, S. R. (2016). The role of familiarity for representations in norm-based face space. *PloS One, 11*(5), e0155380. https://doi.org/10.1371/journal.pone.0155380

Felisberti, F. M. (2022). Experiences of ugliness in nature and urban environments. *Empirical Studies of the Arts, 40*(2), 192–208. https://doi.org/10.1177/02762374211001798

Felisbino-Mendes, M. S., Matozinhos, F. P., Miranda, J. J., Villamor, E., & Velasquez-Melendez, G. (2014). Maternal obesity and fetal deaths: results from the Brazilian cross-sectional demographic health survey, 2006. *BMC Pregnancy and Childbirth, 14*(1), 1–19. https://doi.org/10.1186/1471-2393-14-5

Feng L. F. (2020). Characteristics and emerging trends in modern aesthetic medicine. *Chinese Medical Journal, 133*(6), 741–742. https://doi.org/10.1097/CM9.0000000000000679

Foo, Y. Z., Simmons, L. W., & Rhodes, G. (2017). Predictors of facial attractiveness and health in humans. *Scientific Reports, 7*(1), 1–12. https://doi.org/10.1038/srep39731

Gangestad, S. W. (2022). Developmental instability, fluctuating asymmetry, and human psychological science. *Emerging Topics in Life Sciences, 6*(3), 311–322. https://doi.org/10.1042/ETLS20220025

Garcia, L. (2015). The aesthetics of wabi-sabi: beautiful imperfection. *Philosophia: International Journal of Philosophy (Philippine e-journal) 16*(1), 1–18.

Gelepithis, M., & Giani, M. (2022). Inclusion without solidarity: education, economic security, and attitudes toward redistribution. *Political Studies, 70*(1), 45–61. https://doi.org/10.1177/0032321720933082

Gilbert, S. F. (2000). *Developmental Biology*. 6th edition. Sinauer Associates.

Gorbunova, V., Seluanov, A., Mao, Z., & Hine, C. (2007). Changes in DNA repair during aging. *Nucleic Acids Research, 35*(22), 7466–7474. https://doi.org/10.1093/nar/gkm756

Grammer, K., & Thornhill, R. (1994). Human (homo sapiens) facial attractiveness and sexual selection: the role of symmetry and averageness. *Journal of Comparative Psychology, 108*(3), 233–242.

Gray, A. W., & Boothroyd, L. G. (2012). Female facial appearance and health. *Evolutionary Psychology, 10*(1), 66–77. https://doi.org/10.1177/147470491201000108

Hahn, K. A., Hatch, E. E., Rothman, K. J., Mikkelsen, E. M., Brogly, S. B., Sørensen, H. T., Riis, A. H., & Wise, L. A. (2014). Body size and risk of spontaneous abortion among Danish pregnancy planners. *Pediatric and Perinatal Epidemiology, 28*(5), 412–423. https://doi.org/10.1111/ppe.12142

Harper, D. (2023). *Online Etymology Dictionary. Beauty*. Retrieved Dec. 22, 2023, from https://www.etymonline.com/search?q=beauty

Haselberger, H. (1961). Method of studying ethnological art. *Current Anthropology, 2*(4), 341–384.

Haughton N. (2004). Perceptions of beauty in Renaissance art. *Journal of Cosmetic Dermatology, 3*(4), 229–233. https://doi.org/10.1111/j.1473-2130.2004.00142.x

He, D., Workman, C. I., Kenett, Y. N., He, X., & Chatterjee, A. (2021). The effect of aging on facial attractiveness: an empirical and computational investigation. *Acta Psychologica, 219*, 103385. https://doi.org/10.1016/j.actpsy.2021.103385

Hoffmann, D. L., Standish, C. D., García-Diez, M., Pettitt, P. B., Milton, J. A., Zilhão, J., Alcolea-González, J. J., Cantalejo-Duarte, P., Collado, H., de Balbín, R., Lorblanchet, M., Ramos-Muñoz, J., Weniger, G. C., & Pike, A. W. G. (2018). U-Th dating of carbonate crusts reveals Neandertal origin of Iberian cave art. *Science (New York, N.Y.), 359*(6378), 912–915. https://doi.org/10.1126/science.aap7778

Hornby, A. S. (ed.) (2011*). Oxford Advanced Learner's Dictionary of Current English*. Oxford University Press.

Hubbard, J. S., Rohrmann, S., Landis, P., Metter, E. J., Muller, D. C., Andres, R., Carter, H., & Platz, E. A. (2004). Association of prostate cancer risk with insulin, glucose, and anthropometry in the Baltimore longitudinal study of aging. *Urology, 63*(2), 253–258. https://doi.org/10.1016/j.urology.2003.09.060

Hung, S. M., Nieh, C. H., & Hsieh, P. J. (2016). Unconscious processing of facial attractiveness: invisible attractive faces orient visual attention. *Scientific Reports, 6*, 37117. https://doi.org/10.1038/srep37117

Hwang, K., & Park, C. Y. (2021). The divine proportion: origins and usage in plastic surgery. *Plastic and Reconstructive Surgery. Global Open, 9*(2), e3419. https://doi.org/10.1097/GOX.0000000000003419

Jackson, M., Walker, S., Simpson, C. M., Mcfarlane-Anderson, N., Bennett, F. I., Coard, K. C. M., Aiken, W., Tulloch, T., Paul, T., & Wan, R. L. (2010). Body size and risk of prostate cancer in Jamaican men. *Cancer Causes & Control, 21*(6), 909–917. https://doi.org/10.1007/s10552-010-9520-y

Jacobsen T. (2010). Beauty and the brain: culture, history and individual differences in aesthetic appreciation. *Journal of Anatomy, 216*(2), 184–191. https://doi.org/10.1111/j.1469-7580.2009.01164.x

Jasienska, G., Lipson, S. F., Ellison, P. T., Thune, I., & Ziomkiewicz, A. (2006). Symmetrical women have higher potential fertility. *Evolution and Human Behavior, 27*(5), 390–400. https://doi.org/10.1016/j.evolhumbehav.2006.01.001

Jones, A. L., & Jäger, B. (2019). Biological bases of beauty revisited: the effect of symmetry, averageness, and sexual dimorphism on female facial attractiveness. *Symmetry, 11*(2), 279. https://doi.org/10.3390/sym11020279

Jones, B. C., Little, A. C., Burt, D. M., & Perrett, D. I. (2004). When facial attractiveness is only skin deep. *Perception, 33*(5), 569–576. https://doi.org/10.1068/p3463

Katsilambros, N., Georgiadis, E., Aliferis, C. F., Papandreou, L., Triantaphyllou, D., Kouroutis, S., Grigoriadis, N., & Tzavaras, A. (1993). Serum lipids and arterial blood pressure in relation to waist-to-hip ratio in young males. *The American Journal of Clinical Nutrition, 57*(5), 697–698. https://doi.org/10.1093/ajcn/57.5.697

Kiiski, H. S., Cullen, B., Clavin, S. L., & Newell, F. N. (2016). Perceptual and social attributes underlining age-related preferences for faces. *Frontiers in Human Neuroscience, 10*, 437. https://doi.org/10.3389/fnhum.2016.00437

Kirwan, J. (2023). To what does the word 'Beauty' refer? *ESPES. The Slovak Journal of Aesthetics, 12*(2), 13–27. https://doi.org/10.5281/zenodo.10491689

Králik, Ľ. (2015). *Stručný etymologický slovník slovenčiny*. [A Concise Etymological Dictionary of Slovak]. VEDA, vydavateľstvo SAV; Jazykovedný ústav Ľudovíta Štúra SAV.

Kuppens, T., & Spears, R. (2014). You don't have to be well-educated to be an aversive racist, but it helps. *Social Science Research, 45*, 211–223. https://doi.org/10.1016/j.ssresearch.2014.01.006

Kuraguchi, K., Taniguchi, K., & Ashida, H. (2015). The impact of baby schema on perceived attractiveness, beauty, and cuteness in female adults. *SpringerPlus, 4*(1), 164. https://doi.org/10.1186/s40064-015-0940-8

Lassek, W. D., & Gaulin, S. J. C. (2008). Waist-hip ratio and cognitive ability: is gluteofemoral fat a privileged store of neurodevelopmental resources? *Evolution and Human Behavior, 29*(1), 26–34. https://doi.org/10.1016/j.evolhumbehav.2007.07.00

Li, R., & Zhang, J. (2020). Review of computational neuroaesthetics: bridging the gap between neuroaesthetics and computer science. *Brain Informatics, 7*(1), 16. https://doi.org/10.1186/s40708-020-00118-w

Liang, X., Zebrowitz, L. A., & Zhang, Y. (2010). Neural activation in the „reward circuit" shows a nonlinear response to facial attractiveness. *Social Neuroscience, 5*(3), 320–334. https://doi.org/10.1080/17470911003619916

Liddell, H., G., & Scott, R. (1940). *A Greek-English Lexicon; Machine Readable Text.* Trustees of Tufts University.

Little, A. (2014). Domain specificity in human symmetry preferences: Symmetry is most pleasant when looking at human faces. *Symmetry, 6*(2), 222–233. https://doi.org/10.3390/sym6020222

Little, A. C., Debruine, L. M., & Jones, B. C. (2011b). Exposure to visual cues of pathogen contagion changes preferences for masculinity and symmetry in opposite-sex faces. *Proceedings of the Royal Society of London B: Biological Sciences, 278*(1714), 2032–2039. https://doi.org/10.1098/rspb.2010.1925

Little, A. C., Jones, B. C., & Debruine, L. M. (2011a). Facial attractiveness: evolutionary based research. *Philosophical Transactions of the Royal Society of London. Series B, Biological Sciences, 366*(1571), 1638–1659. https://doi.org/10.1098/rstb.2010.0404

Little, A. C., Jones, B. C., Debruine, L. M., & Feinberg, D. R. (2008). Symmetry and sexual dimorphism in human faces: interrelated preferences suggest both signal quality. *Behavioral Ecology, 19*(4), 902–908. https://doi.org/10.1093/beheco/arn049

Little, A. C., Jones, B. C., Feinberg, D. R., & Perrett, D. I. (2014). Men's strategic preferences for femininity in female faces. *British Journal of Psychology, 105*(3), 364–381. https://doi.org/10.1111/bjop.12043

Livshits, G., & Kobyliansky, E. (1984). Biochemical heterozygosity as a predictor of developmental homeostasis in man. *Annals of Human Genetics, 48*(2), 173–184. https://doi.org/10.1111/j.1469-1809.1984.tb01012.x

Lloyd, D. R. (2010). Symmetry and Beauty in Plato. *Symmetry, 2*(2), 455–465. https://doi.org/10.3390/sym2020455

Machilsen, B., Pauwels, M., & Wagemans, J. (2009) The role of vertical mirror symmetry in visualshape detection. *Journal of Vision, 9*(12), 1–11. https://doi.org/10.1167/9.12.11

Maisey, D. S., Vale, E. L., Cornelissen, P., & Tovée, M. J. (1999). Characteristics of male attractiveness for women. *The Lancet, 353*(9163), 1500. https://doi.org/10.1016/s0140-6736(99)00438-9

Makin, A. D. J., Pecchinenda, A., & Bertamini, M. (2012). Implicit affective evaluation of visual symmetry. *Emotion, 12*(5), 1021–1030. https://doi.org/10.1037/a0026924

Manning, J. T., Scutt, D., & Lewis-Jones, D. I. (1998). Developmental stability, ejaculate size, and sperm quality in men. *Evolution and Human Behavior, 19*(5), 273–282. https://doi.org/10.1016/S1090-5138(98)00024-5

Marcinkowska, U. M., Jasienska, G., & Prokop, P. (2018). A comparison of masculinity facial preference among naturally cycling, pregnant, lactating, and post-menopausal women. *Archives of Sexual Behavior, 47*(5), 1367–1374. https://doi.org/10.1007/s10508-017-1093-3

Martin-Loeches, M., Hernández-Tamames, J. A., Martín, A., & Urrutia, M. (2014). Beauty and ugliness in the bodies and faces of others: an fMRI study of person esthetic judgement. *Neuroscience, 277*, 486–497. https://doi.org/10.1016/j.neuroscience.2014.07.040

Maynard, S., Fang, E. F., Scheibye-Knudsen, M., Croteau, D. L., & Bohr, V. A. (2015). DNA damage, DNA repair, aging, and neurodegeneration. *Cold Spring Harbor Perspectives in Medicine, 5*(10), a025130. https://doi.org/10.1101/cshperspect.a025130

McIntosh, C. (ed.) (2013). *Cambridge Advanced Learner's Dictionary*. Cambridge University Press.

Menninghaus, W., Wagner, V., Kegel, V., Knoop, C. A., & Schlotz, W. (2019). Beauty, elegance, grace, and sexiness compared. *PloS One, 14*(6), e0218728. https://doi.org/10.1371/journal.pone.0218728

Mirfazeli, F. S., Lai, M. C., Memari, A., Rajab, A., Shafizadeh, M., Zarei, S., Shariat, S. V., Fashi, M. H., Barzegary, E., & Vahabie, A. H. (2021). Short-term and long-term mate preference in men and women in an Iranian population. *Scientific Reports, 11*(1), 20752. https://doi.org/10.1038/s41598-021-99653-7

Mitteroecker, P., Windhager, S., Müller, G. B., & Schaefer, K. (2015). The morphometrics of "masculinity" in human faces. *Plos One, 10*(2), e0118374. https://doi.org/10.1371/journal.pone.0118374

Møller, A. P. (1990). Fluctuating asymmetry in male sexual ornaments may reliably reveal male quality. *Animal Behaviour, 40*(6), 1185–1187. https://doi.org/10.1016/S0003-3472(05)80187-3

Møller, A. P. (1997). Developmental stability and fitness: a review. *The American Naturalist, 149*(5), 916–932. https://doi.org/10.1086/286030

Møller, A. P., Soler, M., & Thornhill, R. (1995). Breast asymmetry, sexual selection, and human reproductive success. *Ethology and Sociobiology, 16*(3), 207–219. https://doi.org/10.1016/0162-3095(95)00002-3

Montgomery Sklar E. (2015). Body image, weight, and self-concept in men. *American Journal of Lifestyle Medicine, 11*(3), 252–258. https://doi.org/10.1177/1559827615594351

Mudrik, L., Deouell, L. Y., & Lamy, D. (2011). Scene congruency biases binocular rivalry. *Consciousness and Cognition, 20*(3), 756–767. https://doi.org/10.1016/j.concog.2011.01.001

Mühlenbeck, C., Liebal, K., Pritsch, C., & Jacobsen, T. (2016). Differences in the visual perception of symmetric patterns in orangutans (Pongo Pygmaeus Abelii) and two human cultural groups: a comparative eye-tracking study. Frontiers in *Psychology, 7*. https://doi.org/10.3389/fpsyg.2016.00408

Musicco Nombela, D. (2024). What is beauty in the 21st century? *Communication and Man, 20*, 13–20. https://doi.org/10.32466/eufv-cyh.2024.20.830.13-20

Nisanyan, S. (2011). *Sözlerin Soyağacı Çağdaş Türkçenin Kökenbilim Sözlüğü*. Everest Yayınları.

Nisbett, R. E., & Wilson, T. D. (1977). The halo effect: Evidence for unconscious alteration of judgments. *Journal of Personality and Social Psychology, 35*(4), 250–256. https://doi.org/10.1037/0022-3514.35.4.250

Nisbett, R. E., & Wilson, T. D. (1977). The halo effect: evidence for unconscious alteration of judgments. *Journal of Personality and Social Psychology, 35*(4), 250–256. https://doi.org/10.1037/0022-3514.35.4.250

Osgood, C. E. (1957). Measurement of meaning. *Psychological Bulletin, 54*(4), pp. 390–407.

Osgood, Ch. E., Suci, G., & Tannenbaum, P. (1957). *The Measurement of Meaning*. University of Illinois Press.

Pawlowski, B. (2001). The evolution of gluteal/femoral fat deposits and balance during pregnancy in bipedal homo. *Current Anthropology, 42*(4), 572–574. http://www.jstor.org/stable/10.1086/322548

Pazhoohi, F., Garza, R., & Kingstone, A. (2023). The interacting effects of height and shoulder-to-hip ratio on perceptions of attractiveness, masculinity, and fighting ability: experimental design and ecological validity considerations. *Archives of Sexual Behavior, 52*(1), 301–314. https://doi.org/10.1007/s10508-022-02416-2

Perrett, D. I. (2010). *In Your Face*. Palgrave Macmillan.

Pfeifer, W. (1993). Etymologisches Wörterbuch des Deutschen. Digitalisierte und von Wolfgang Pfeifer überarbeitete Version im Digitalen Wörterbuch der deutschen Sprache. Retrieved Jan. 12, 2024, from https://www.dwds.de/wb/wb-etymwb

Pflüger, L. S., Oberzaucher, E., Katina, S., Holzleitner, I. J., & Grammer, K. (2012). Cues to fertility: perceived attractiveness and facial shape predict reproductive success. *Evolution and Human Behavior, 33*(6), 708–714. https://doi.org/10.1016/j.evolhumbehav.2012.05.00

Pitcher, D., Walsh, V., & Duchaine, B. (2011). Transcranial magnetic stimulation studies of face processing. In A. J. Calder, G. Rhodes, M. H. Johnson, & J. V. Haxby (eds.) *The Oxford Handbook of Face Perception* (pp. 367–386), Oxford University Press.

Platón. (1979). *Dialógy o kráse*. [Dialogues about Beauty]. Odeon.

Plotinus, B. S. (2016). *The Six Enneads*. Create Space Independent Publishing Platform.

Pradier, A. (2022). Free beauty and functional perspective in medieval aesthetics. *Religions. 13*(2), 125. https://doi.org/10.3390/rel13020125

Rahal, D., Fales, M. R., Haselton, M. G., Slavich, G. M., & Robles, T. F. (2021). Cues of social status: associations between attractiveness, dominance, and status. *Evolutionary Psychology : An International Journal of Evolutionary Approaches to Psychology and Behavior, 19*(0), 14747049211056160. https://doi.org/10.1177/14747049211056160

Rahman, S. Z. (2003). Were the "Dark Ages" really dark?. *Grey Matter (The Co-curricular Journal of Jawaharlal Nehru Medical College)*, Aligarh Muslim University, 7–10.

Rakhmatova, M. M. (2019). Linguistic features of the concept "beauty" in English, Uzbek and Tajik national cultures. *ISJ Theoretical & Applied Science, 10*(78), 764–770. https://dx.doi.org/10.15863/TAS.2019.10.78.145

Reber, R. (2002). Reasons for the preference for symmetry. *Behavioral and Brain Sciences, 25*(3), 415–416. https://doi.org/10.1017/S0140525X02350076

Reber, R., Schwarz, N., & Winkielman, P. (2004). Processing fluency and aesthetic pleasure: is beauty in the perceiver's processing experience? *Personality and Social Psychology Review, 8*(4), 364–382. https://doi.org/10.1207/s15327957pspr0804_3

Redies, C. (2015). Combining universal beauty and cultural context in a unifying model of visual aesthetic experience. *Frontiers in Human Neuroscience, 9*, 218. https://doi.org/10.3389/fnhum.2015.00218

Rejzek, J. (2001). Český etymologický slovník. [Czech Etymological Dictionary]. Leda.

Rhodes, G. (2006). The evolutionary psychology of facial beauty. *Annual Review of Psychology, 57*, 199–226. https://doi.org/10.1146/annurev.psych.57.102904.190208

Rhodes, G., Chan, J., Zebrowitz, L. A., & Simmons, L. W. (2003). Does sexual dimorphism in human faces signal health? *Proceedings of the Royal Society B. Biological Sciences, 270*(1), 83–95. https://doi.org/10.1098/rsbl.2003.0023

Rhodes, G., Yoshikawa, S., Clark, A., Lee, K., McKay, R., & Akamatsu, S. (2001). Attractiveness of facial averageness and symmetry in non-Western cultures: in search of biologically based standards of beauty. *Perception, 30*(5), 611–625. https://doi.org/10.1068/p3123

Riji, H. M. (2006). Beauty or health? A personal view. *Malaysian Family Physician: The Official Journal of the Academy of Family Physicians of Malaysia, 1*(1), 42–44.

Rivera-Garrido, N. (2022). Can education reduce traditional gender role attitudes? *Economics of Education Review, 89*, 102261. https://doi.org/10.1016/j.econodurov.2022.102261

Salehi, P., Azadeh, N., Beigi, N., & Farzin, M. (2019). Influence of age on perception of best esthetical profile. *Journal of Dentistry (Shiraz, Iran), 20*(1), 16–23. https://doi.org/10.30476/DENTJODS.2019.44558

Salusso-Deonier, C. J., Markee, N. L., & Pedersen, E. L. (1993). Gender differences in the evaluation of physical attractiveness ideals for male and female body builds. *Perceptual and Motor Skills, 76*(3), 1155–1167. https://doi.org/10.2466/pms.1993.76.3c.115

Scheib, J. E., Gangestad, S. W., & Thornhill, R. (1999). Facial attractiveness, symmetry and cues of good genes. *Proceedings. Biological Sciences, 266*(1431), 1913–1917. https://doi.org/10.1098/rspb.1999.0866.

Schiller, J., Ch., F. (1943). *Schillers Werke, Nationalausgabe*, Julius Petersen et al. (eds.), 43 vols., Hermann Böhlaus Nachfolger.

Schiller, J., Ch., F. (1793/2003). Kallias or Concerning Beauty: Letters to Gottfried Körner, Stefan Bird-Polan (trans.), in J. M. Bernstein (ed.), *Classic and Romantic German Aesthetics*, Cambridge University Press. pp. 145–183.

Schindler, I., Hosoya, G., Menninghaus, W., Beermann, U., Wagner, V., Eid, M., & Scherer, K. R. (2017). Measuring aesthetic emotions: a review of the literature and a new assessment tool. *PloS One, 12*(6), e0178899. https://doi.org/10.1371/journal.pone.0178899

Scott, R. (2022). Does university make you more liberal? Estimating the within-individual effects of higher education on political values. *Electoral Studies, 77*, 102471. https://doi.org/10.1016/j.electstud.2022.102471

Scruton, R. (2011). *Beauty: A Very Short Introduction.* Oxford University Press.

Shackelford, T. K., & Larsen, R. J. (1997). Facial asymmetry as an indicator of psychological, emotional, and physiological distress. *Journal of Personality and Social Psychology, 72*(2), 456–466. https://doi.org/10.1037/0022-3514.72.2.456

Shi, A., Huo, F., & Hou, G. (2021). Effects of design aesthetics on the perceived value of a product. *Frontiers in Psychology, 12*, 670800. https://doi.org/10.3389/fpsyg.2021.670800

Sibbald, B. (2016). End coming for misunderstood CMA House. *CMAJ : Canadian Medical Association journal = journal de l'Association medicale canadienne, 188*(9), 642–644. https://doi.org/10.1503/cmaj.109-5279

Sidhu, D. M., McDougall, K. H., Jalava, S. T., & Bodner, G. E. (2018). Prediction of beauty and liking ratings for abstract and representational paintings using subjective and objective measures. *PloS One, 13*(7), e0200431. https://doi.org/10.1371/journal.pone.0200431

Simmons, L. W., Rhodes, G., Peters, M., & Koehlerb, N. (2004). Are human preferences for facial symmetry focused on signals of developmental instability? *Behavioral Ecology, 15*(5), 864–871. https://doi.org/10.1093/beheco/arh099

Singh D. (2002). Female mate value at a glance: relationship of waist-to-hip ratio to health, fecundity and attractiveness. *Neuro Endocrinology Letters, 23*(Suppl. 4), 81–91.

Singh, D. (1993). Adaptive significance of female physical attractiveness: role of waist-to-hip ratio. *Journal of Personality and Social Psychology, 65*(2), 293–307. https://doi.org/10.1037/0022-3514.65.2.293

Singh, D., & Singh, D. (2011). Shape and significance of feminine beauty: an evolutionary perspective. *Sex Roles, 64*(9), 723–731. https://doi.org/10.1007/s11199-011-9938-z

Sorokowski, P. (2010). Did Venus have long legs? Beauty standards from various historical periods reflected in works of art. *Perception, 39*(10), 1427–1430. https://doi.org/10.1068/p6621

Sugiyama, L. S. (2004). Is beauty in the context-sensitive adaptations of the beholder? *Evolution and Human Behavior, 25*(1), 51–62. https://doi.org/10.1016/s1090-5138(03)00083-7

Synonymický slovník slovenčiny [Slovak Thesaurus]. (2004). Jazykovedný ústav Ľ. Štúra SAV. https://slovnik.juls.savba.sk/?w=kr%C3%A1sa&s=exact&c=I72e&cs=&d=sss#

Tambe, D. B., Phadke, A. V., Kharche, J. S., & Joshi, A. R. (2010). Correlation of blood pressure with body mass index (BMI) and waist to hip ratio (WHR) in middle aged men. *Internet Journal of Medical Update, 5*(2), 26–30.

Tangney, J. P., Stuewig, J., & Mashek, D. J. (2007). Moral emotions and moral behavior. *Annual Review of Psychology, 58,* 345–372. https://doi.org/10.1146/annurev.psych.56.091103.070145

Tatarkiewicz, W. (1980). Beauty: history of the concept. In *A History of Six Ideas*. Melbourne International Philosophy Series, vol. 5. Springer (pp. 121–152). Dordrecht. https://doi.org/10.1007/978-94-009-8805-7_5

Thesaurus (2024). *Beauty*. Retrieved Feb. 18, 2024 from https://www.thesaurus.com/browse/beauty

Tsukiura, T., & Cabeza, R. (2011). Shared brain activity for aesthetic and moral judgments: implications for the Beauty-is-Good stereotype. *Social Cognitive and Affective Neuroscience, 6*(1), 138–148. https://doi.org/10.1093/scan/nsq025

Ulger, K. (2016). The creative training in the visual arts education. *Thinking Skills and Creativity, 19,* 73–87. https://doi.org/10.1016/j.tsc.2015.10.007

Underwood, G. (2005). Eye fixations on pictures of natural scenes: getting the gist and identifying the components. In G. Underwood (ed.), *Cognitive Processes in Eye Guidance* (pp. 163–187). Oxford University Press.

Vaidyanathan, B., Haraburda, B., & Jacobi, C. J. (2023). Beauty in biology: an empirical assessment. *Journal of Biosciences, 48,* 15.

Vandiver, P. B., Soffer, O., Klima, B., & Svoboda, J. (1989). The origins of ceramic technology at Dolni Věstonice, Czechoslovakia. *Science (New York, N.Y.), 246*(4933), 1002–1008. https://doi.org/10.1126/science.246.4933.1002

Vavrová, M., & Démuthová, S. (2021). Interpohlavné rozdiely v konotátoch pojmu krása. [Intersexual Differences in the Connotations of the Concept of Beauty]. In Z. Rojková, & D. Kochanová, (eds.), *Kondášove dni 2021 : zborník vedeckých recenzovaných príspevkov z konferencie* [Kondáš Days 2021: Proceedings of Scientific Peer-Reviewed Contributions from the Conference] (pp. 69–76). Katedra psychológie FF UCM v Trnave.

Vladimirova, S. V., Aryabkina, I. V., Beregovaya, E. B., Stukalova, O. V., & Alekseeva, L. L. (2019). Art education and its impact effects on modern students. In S. K. Lo (ed.), *Education Environment for the Information Age, vol. 69. European Proceedings of Social and Behavioural Sciences* (pp. 57–66). Future Academy. https://doi.org/10.15405/epsbs.2019.09.02.8

Vrábel, P. (2005). *Heuristika a metodológia matematiky*. [Heuristics and Methodology of Mathematics]. FPV Univerzita Konštantína Filozofa.

World Health Organization: WHO. (2008). *Waist circumference and waist-hip ratio report of a WHO expert consultation Geneva*, 8–11 December 2008. World Health Organization.

World Health Organization: WHO. (2022). *Ageing and health*. www.who.int. Retrieved Feb. 20, 2024 from https://www.who.int/news-room/fact-sheets/detail/ageing-and-health

Wulff, D. U., Hills, T. T., & Mata, R. (2022). Structural differences in the semantic networks of younger and older adults. *Scientific Reports, 12*(1), 21459. https://doi.org/10.1038/s41598-022-11698-4

Yang, T., Formuli, A., Paolini, M., & Zeki, S. (2022). The neural determinants of beauty. *The European Journal of Neuroscience, 55*(1), 91–106. https://doi.org/10.1111/ejn.15543

Yarosh, D. B. (2019). Perception and deception: human beauty and the brain. *Behavioral Sciences, 9*(4), 34. https://doi.org/10.3390/bs9040034

Yu, K., & Blake, R. (1992). Do recognizable figures enjoy an advantage in binocular rivalry? *Journal of Experimental Psychology: Human Perception and Performance, 18*(4), 1158–1173. https://doi.org/10.1037/0096-1523.18.4.1158

Yuan, R., Yang, M., & Stapleton, P. (2020). Enhancing undergraduates' critical thinking through research engagement: a practitioner research approach. *Thinking Skills and Creativity, 38*. https://doi.org/10.1016/j.tsc.2020.100737

Zanchi, G. (2020). *La Bellezza Complice*. Rubbettine Editore.

Zeki, S., Chén, O. Y., & Romaya, J. P. (2018) The biological basis of mathematical beauty. *Frontiers in Human Neuroscience, 12*, 467. https://10.3389/fnhum.2018.00467

Zelazniewicz, A., Nowak-Kornicka, J., Zbyrowska, K., & Pawłowski, B. (2021). Predicted reproductive longevity and women's facial attractiveness. *Plos One, 16*(3), e0248344. https://doi.org/10.1371/journal.pone.0248344

Zhang, X., Gao, Y., & Rashid, A. (2005). Body mass index (BMI), waist to hip ratio (WHR) and risk of biliary tract cancers: a population – based case – control study in Shanghai, China. *Chinese Journal of Clinical Oncology, 2*(1), 505–510. https://doi.org/10.1007/bf0273974

Zheng, W., Luo, T., Hu, C. P., & Peng, K. (2018). Glued to which face? Attentional priority effect of female babyface and male mature face. *Frontiers in Psychology, 9*, 286. https://doi.org/10.3389/fpsyg.2018.00286

Admiration and Disgust
Social and Moral Emotions
of Admiration and Disgust

Renáta Kišoňová

> *"What does that mean-, admire'?"*
> *"To admire means that you regard me as the handsomest, the best-dressed, the richest, and the most intelligent man on this planet."*
> *"But you are the only man on your planet!"*
> *"Do me this kindness. Admire me just the same."*
> *"I admire you,"* said the little prince, shrugging his shoulders slightly, *"but what is there in that to interest you so much".*
>
> Antoine de Saint Exupéry, Little Prince

An Introduction

Research on human emotionality has been stimulating for centuries, while in recent decades it has moved from the exclusive domain of psychology and philosophy to an increasingly interdisciplinary investigation, which is based on the current results of brain research, neuroscience, anthropology, sociology, evolutionarily oriented sciences (evolutionary biology, evolutionary psychology, evolutionary anthropology, and so on) and cognitive sciences. And although science has now more or less broadly mapped the functioning of human emotions in terms of brain processes (Gray & McNaughton, 2003; Lee & Siegle, 2009; Pessoa, 2013), body expressions and manifestations (especially the face, which first reflects our emotionality (Darwin, 2009; Ekman, 1972, 2015; Simon, 2003; Prasanthi & Prakash, 2020)), the area of the meaning of emotions for the area of morality, or for the area of socialization of an individual, remains largely unexplored or offers contradictory hypotheses. In the following text, I will focus on the meaning of the emotions of admiration and disgust. In some previous texts, I have defined them as opposite each other, or as almost oppositely experienced emotions (Kišoňová, 2021; Kišoňová 2022; Kišoňová, 2023), and in the following text I will look in more details at the possibilities and limits of how to perceive the emotions of admiration and disgust as opposites. The study will also include the results of a questionnaire survey, where

I asked students about the emotions of disgust and admiration. The structure of the text will be as follows: first of all, I will present significant philosophical and scientific approaches to the emotions of admiration and disgust (or to grasping emotionality in general), Aristotle, René Descartes, Charles Darwin, and Jonathan Haidt. Then I will focus on the terminology (ethymology, synonyms, opposites, etc.) and on these two emotions experienced in everyday life and in public space, in the city, and in nature.

I will end the introduction of the text with a longer quote about the color of emotions, which I find very relevant: "[E]motions are often compared to the colors of things. Although emotionality colors the lived experience, gives it a special and subjectively specific character, helps us identify it personally or establish a relationship with it, but at the same time it is also what is unimportant to many things and experiences. If we want to use a chair, it hardly matters what color it is. In most cases, the color of things does not change (does not add or take away from) their function, structure, essence or price. And although there are objects, symptoms or phenomena where the color of the properties or manifestations really matters... in most cases we believe that colors... are just a kind of unimportant property – a case of subjective experience from which we can safely abstract" (Démuth, 2019, p. 11). In the following text, I will try to show the color shades of the emotions of disgust and admiration.

Considering the Emotions of Disgust and Admiration in the History of Philosophy

Although admiration and disgust represent basic emotions, in the history of philosophical writing, various expressions have appeared, which the authors grasped and, as I will show below, they often used them in different meanings.

First of all, let me mention Aristotle and his understanding of emotions. He preferred the term *pathos*[5] (greek pathé) for emo-

---

5 Aristotle characterized in The Nicomachean Ethics pathē as "feelings accompanied by pleasure or pain", mentionning appetite, anger, fear, trust, envy, joy, love,

tion. It makes emotions more passive states, paths are primarily reactions found in the embodied animal to the external world, similar to sensations (Aristotle, 2009; Aristotle, 2013). Aristotle considered emotions to be a kind of movement, since their causes lie outside the animal that experiences them. The main Aristotele question arises whether and to what extent we can control them. He presented the basic emotions of anger, love, hate, meekness, fear, courage, shame, kindness, compassion, envy, and rivalry in the 2nd book of *Rhetoric* in relation to the rhetorician's personality. He does not interpret the emotion of disgust, nor does he use this term in *Rhetoric*; he interprets emotion of *cataphronesis*, contempt, which may be the closest to social emotion of disgust (Aristotle, 2013). This is a question addressed in several different ways by the most important Aristotelian texts on the path available to later ancient and medieval authors: *Nicomachean Ethics* and *Rhetoric*. Each work presents a list of emotions, although where the *Nicomachean Ethics* offers up to 11, the Rhetoric offers a total of 14. They also differ in their goals and meaning: the *Nicomachean Ethics* deals with the place of the journey within the economy of action according to our habits and desires, which are moderated reason, while Rhetoric is about arousing and directing the way in the context of creating persuasion. In both cases, however, the path is considered amenable to rational influence and voluntary action, although not directly subject to choice (Aristotle, 2013; Aristotle, 2009).

Descartes and the Wonder as the Emotion Closest to Admiration

Descartes not only had a theory of passions but also one that deserves a place among contemporary debates on emotion (Franco, 2006). Descartes defined passions: "The passions that are aroused

---

hatred, desire, imitation, and regret as examples (Aristotle, 2009). It will be easiest to regard pathos in Aristotle´s concept as more or less equivalent to desire or appetite in a broader sense.

in us by the objects that stimulate the senses aren't different for every difference among the objects, but only corresponding to differences in how the objects can harm or benefit us, or more generally have importance for us. What the passions do for us consists solely in this: they dispose our soul to want the things that nature decides are useful to us, and to persist in this volition; and the agitation of the spirits that normally causes the passions also disposes the body to move in ways that help to bring about those useful things. That's why a list of the passions requires only an orderly examination of all the various ways – ways that are important to us – in which our senses can be stimulated by their objects. Now I shall list all the principal passions according to the order in which they can thus be found" (Descartes, 1989, p. 17). When our first encounter with any object surprises us and we find it different from what we formerly knew or from what we supposed it should be, this brings it about that we wonder and are astonished at it. "All this can happen before we know whether the object is beneficial to us, so I regard wonder as the first of all the passions. It has no opposite, because if the object before us has nothing surprising about it, it doesn't stir us in any way and we consider it without passion. Esteem (with generosity or pride), and contempt (with humility or abjectness). Wonder is joined to either esteem or contempt, depending on whether we wonder at how (metaphorically speaking) big the objects or at how small. So we can esteem ourselves, giving rise to the passion of magnanimity or pride, and the corresponding behaviour; or contemn ourselves, giving rise to the passion of humility or abjectness, and the corresponding behaviour" (Descartes, 1989, p.18). Descartes did not specifically thematize the emotion of admiration; his understanding of esteem and wonder is perhaps the closest to admiration. Similarly, with disgust, Descartes talks about contempt, which can be seen as a concept close to disgust.

Charles Darwin's Understanding of Emotions

Darwin treated the emotions as separate discrete entities, or modules, such as anger, fear, disgust, joy, and so on (Ekman, 2009).

Darwin proposed that facial expressions of emotions are universal (Darwin, 2020) and gestures are culture-specific conventions (Darwin, 2020).[6] Emotions are not unique to humans but may be found in many other species according to him (bees, roosters, dogs, cats, horses, and other primates). Compared to other emotions, admiration was given a very brief reflection by Darwin. He characterized the emotion of admiration in just a few sentences: "Admiration. Little needs to be said about this emotion. Admiration probably lies in surprise combined with some pleasantness and a feeling of approval. During the experience of vivid admiration, the eyes are open and the eyebrows are raised, expressionless as during simple astonishment, and the mouth is spread into a smile instead of being fully opened" (Darwin 2020, p. 229). Darwin characterizes the emotion of wonder more extensively, which he says has similar physiological reactions to admiration (e.g., acceleration of heart activity and thus also breathing). With concentrated amazement (even admiration) of someone or something, we forget about all the organs of the body; we even neglect them according to Darwin (Darwin, 2020). Darwin investigated the manifestations and reasons for experiencing disgust in more detail than the emotion of admiration. According to him, it refers primarily to the sense of taste and then secondarily to everything that causes a similar sensation through smell, touch, and sight. Physiologically, according to Darwin, we experience it very similarly to the feeling of contempt, i.e. with closed eyelids, possibly averted eyes or even the whole body (we express by this that the despised person or thing is not worthy of our gaze or even our presence and participation). The basis for expressing contempt is the movements around the nose and mouth; if we express them more expressively, we already indicate disgust. "The nose may be slightly turned up, which seems to come from the upper lip being turned up, or the movement may be limited only to wrinkling the nose. The nose is often slightly

---

6 Paul Ekman, analyzing Darwin´s theory, agrees with Darwin: "The same hand movement, for example the first finger touching the thumb to form a circle in the North American 'A-OK' gesture, has a radically different meaning in other countries. Totally different gestures may be used to signal the same message, as in the example of 'good luck' signaled by crossed fingers in North America and thumbs inserted into the fist in Germany. And there are messages for which there is a gesture in one country and no gesture in another country" (Ekman, 2009).

constricted so that the passage is partially closed, which is usually accompanied by a light snort or exhalation (through the nose). All these activities are identical to those we use when we perceive a foul smell and wish to prevent or expel it" (Darwin 2020, p. 202).

Jonathan Haidt's Understanding of Morality of Emotions

Haidt reflected emotions as component features, such as an eliciting event, a facial expression, a physiological change, a phenomenological experience, and a motivation or action tendency following also previous theories and researches (Frijda, 1986; Shweder, 1994). According to his concept of moral emotions, two of those components are useful for identifying the moral emotions, for they are easily linked to the interests of society or of other people: elicitors and action tendencies (Haidt, 2003). Haidt mentioned the first component as disinterested elicitors. "Some emotions, such as fear and happiness, occur primarily when good or bad things happen to the self. They can also occur when good or bad things happen to another person, but such reactions seem to require the self to be related to the other (as when one is happy for a friend's success), or to identify temporarily with the other (as when one fears for the protagonist in a movie). Other emotions can be triggered easily and frequently even when the self has no stake in the triggering event. Simply reading about an injustice, or seeing a photograph of a suffering child, can trigger anger or sympathy. Anger may be most frequently triggered by perceived injustices against the self, and sympathy may be most strongly felt for one's kin, but the point here is that some emotions are easily triggered by triumphs, tragedies, and transgressions that do not directly touch the self, while other emotions are not. The more an emotion tends to be triggered by such disinterested elicitors, the more it can be considered a prototypical moral emotion" (Haidt, 2003, p. 853). The second component, according to Haidt, is pro-social action tendencies. Emotions motivate some sort of action as a response to the eliciting event, although the action is often not taken; the emotion puts the person into a cognitive state in which there is an increased tendency to engage in certain goal-related actions like revenge, affiliation, or comforting and so on (Haidt, 2003; Frijda, 1986). Haidt created a two-dimensional space in which one axis shows the degree to which an emotion can be elicited by situations that do not directly harm or benefit the self and the second axis shows the degree to which an emotion's action tendencies are prosocial (Haidt, 2003). "Each emotion and its many variants can partake to a greater or lesser degree in each of the two features that make an emotion a moral emotion. Anger, for example...in its 'best case' scenario can be felt in disinterested situations, with highly prosocial action tendencies. In other cases... with highly self-interested appraisals and anti-social action tendencies" (Haidt, 2003, p. 853).[7] Jonathan Haidt links similarly emotion of disgust to the realm of morality (Haidt, 2013), arguing that disgust provides us with a valuable warning that we are going too far: the fact is that in this day and age, when anything is permitted, as long as it is done freely, and when our human nature no longer inspires any respect and we look at our body as an instrument of our autonomous rational will, the feeling of repulsion may be the only, last voice that is still heard in defense of the very core of our humanity. Haidt assumed that we always feel moral disgust when we see that someone behaves in such a way that he belongs to the low levels of some imaginary scale of the social dimension (the top belongs to moral perfection, in some concepts to God and gradually descends to people, animals, monsters, and evil spirit up to absolute evil). "When someone robs a bank, they are doing evil and we want them to be punished. But a man who betrays his own parents or forces children into prostitution seems downright repugnant – as if he lacks some basic human feelings. Such actions arouse in us disgust and seem to trigger the same physiology of disgust as, for example, the sight of rats running out of a garbage can" (Haidt, 2013). We do not know when the feeling of disgust was born in our ancestors, but we know that it does not exist in any other animal. Some mammals reject certain food because it doesn't taste good or smells unpleasant, but only humans reject food because it came

---

7 For a contemporary interdisciplinary research of the emotion of anger, see Démuth, 2024.

into contact with someone or something "unclean" or unattractive. We refuse for the same reasons, and if we can't refuse, we at least eliminate staying in spaces that are dirty, smelly, and repel us. We avoid dirty, smelly underpasses, dark, unventilated corners, and places that seem dangerous and repulsive at first glance. I will mention one experimental research presented by Haidt (Haidt, 2013). Respondents were asked to make a moral judgment when the researchers activated an alarm device designed to signal that they were dealing with something disgusting. I will explain in more detail. Alex Jordan, a graduate student at Stanford University, scouted out a crosswalk on campus, stood at it, and asked passersby to fill out a short questionnaire. People were asked to judge four problematic issues, such as a first-cousin marriage or a film studio's decision to release a documentary despite the director's trickery of getting some of the actors to interview them. Alex Jordan was standing in close proximity to the trash that he had emptied earlier. Each time he addressed another respondent, he previously discreetly placed a new plastic bag inside the basket. He prepared special conditions for half of the participants. Before they even approached, he sprayed two doses of spray into the bag, permeating the entire intersection for a few minutes. The second half of the respondents did not spray the spray into the bin. And indeed, people breathing polluted, smelly air judged the given subjects more harshly (Haidt, 2013). Haidt explained this by saying that we use affect as information. When we decide what we want to think about, we look into ourselves and if we experience unpleasant feelings, we associate them with the evaluation of the given problem. Immorality awakens in us a feeling of bodily impurity and disgust.

The Terms "Emotion", "Feeling", and "Affect"

The terms "feeling", "emotion", and "affect" are interchanged in natural language, everyday use, and also in literature. What do we actually mean by emotion and what does the concept of honor mean? Do these terms need to be distinguished, or do they act as synonyms? The usual definition of the term "emotion says" that an emotion is an affective state of consciousness, during which we experience joy, fear, hatred, and the like, while it is a powerful burst of feelings accompanied by physiological changes (crying, trembling, increased temperature, redness, and the like) (Cambridge Dictionary, 1995). The term "sensation" is defined as the ability to perceive touch, a bodily experience not connected to sight, hearing, taste, or smell (feeling of heat, feeling of cold, feeling of pain), and self-awareness (feeling of inferiority). Feeling is a general term for subjective experience, opinion, and the term "emotion" is related to heightened feelings (Cambridge Dictionary, 1995). Passion (desire) represents extremely strong, compelling emotions. Desires are motivations that "drive us to approach certain stimuli in our environment and engage with them in activities that provide us with a relative gain in immediate pleasure (including relief from discomfort)" (Hofmann et al. 2015, p. 62). Definitions of affects by psychologists work with both terms, emotion and feeling. According to their definition, affect means: "[A]ny experience of feeling or emotion, ranging from suffering to elation, from the simplest to the most complex sensations of feeling, and from the most normal to the most pathological emotional reactions. Often described in terms of positive affect or negative affect, both mood and emotion are considered affective states. Along with cognition and conation, affect is one of the three traditionally identified components of the mind" (https://dictionary.apa.org/affect). Attempts at a scientific interpretation of emotion can already be found in Galen (Koukolík, 2012), and Darwin's work The expression of the emotions in man and animals became the starting point for the current investigation of primary emotions. When we move later, to the 20th century, an original approach to the research of emotions and feelings was taken by Antonio Damasio in the 1990s. Damasio's essential insight is that feelings are mental experiences of body states, which arise as the brain interprets emotions; they are themselves physical states arising from the body's responses to external stimuli (Damasio, 2000). The order of such events is: I am threatened, experience fear, and feel horror. He defined feelings as follows: "The essence of a feeling may not be an elusive mental quality attached to an object, but rather the direct perception of a specific landscape: that of the body...I propose that the critical networks on which feelings rely include not only the traditionally acknowledged collection of brain structures known as the limbic system but also some of the brain›s prefrontal cortices, and, most importantly, the brain sectors that map and integrate signals from the body. I conceptualize the essence of feelings as something you and I can see through a window that opens directly onto a continuously updated image of the structure and state of our body... By and large, a feeling is the momentary 'view' of a part of that body landscape" (Damasio, 1994, p. 18-19). Damasio has suggested that consciousness, whether the primitive core consciousness of animals or the "extended" self-conception of humans, requiring autobiographical memory, emerges from emotions and feelings. His insights, dating back to the early 1990s, emerged from a clinical study of brain lesions in patients who were unable to make correct decisions because their emotions were disturbed but whose reason was otherwise unaffected (Damasio, 1994). Emotions are evoked by perceived or imagined stimuli that generate a wide range of physiological responses, body states as Damasio calls them, and they generate sets of mental images associated with body states (Damasio, 1994). If you are, for example, walking in the woods and come across a bear, your perception of the bear is large bulk, possibly moving quickly toward you, will result in a series of physiological changes: your pulse and respiration will quicken, your blood pressure will rise, your pupils will dilate, and adrenaline and other neurotransmitters will be released. Your brain senses these physiological responses, generates a host of mental images associated with this collective body state, and experiences the feeling you know as "fear" (Damasio, 1994). The unconscious physiological responses precede the conscious awareness of the feeling. As Damasio said: "I propose that human reason depends on several brain systems, working in concert across many levels of neuronal organization, rather than on a single brain center. Both 'high-level' and 'low-level' brain regions...cooperate in the making of reason. The lower levels in the neural edifice of reason are the same ones that regulate the processing of emotions and feelings, along with the body functions necessary for an organism's survival. In turn, these lower levels maintain direct and mutual relationships with virtually every body organ, thus placing the body directly within the chain of operations that generate the highest reaches of reasoning, decision-making, and, by extension, social behavior and creativity. Emotion, feeling and biological regulation all play a role in human reason" (Damasio, 1994, p. 17).

The Brain and the Emotions

Let's see what happens to our brain when we experience emotions. When we observe someone who consumes anything and looks disgusted, we assume that the consumed object is disgusting or contaminated, smelly, or not worth eating. What happens in observer´s brain then? The cognitive hypothesis assumes that the processing of the expression in the observed face leads to a conceptual representation of the state of disgust and the result is a decision to not consume the object. Wicker tested a different hypothesis, based on the fact that experiencing disgust from smells or food activates the insula and amygdala. Wicker and colleagues tested whether this was also true when viewing faces representing disgust (Wicker et al., 2013). Wicker and his colleagues used fMRI in their research: they examined the reactions of 14 healthy men, subjecting them to two visual and two olfactory tests. The visual testing was threefold: observation of disgust, observation of delight, and observation of the neutral expression of the individual who sniffed the contents of the bottle. In the olfactory investigation, olfactory stimuli were used that evoked disgust and evoked pleasant feelings. The amygdala was activated by both disgust and pleasant olfactory stimuli. In the insula, these stimuli activated different areas: disgust-evoking cues activated the front part of the insula bilaterally, and the pleasant olfactory stimuli activated rather the back part of the insula only on the right side. During visual testing, the areas of activation of disgust versus a neutral expression of pleasure versus a neutral expression were compared. Activation of the insula was only detected when comparing the activation of the disgust versus the neutral expression. Some insular areas were activated both when comparing the disgust state versus the neutral state, as well as when smelling the stimulus that arouses disgust compared to the calm state (Wicker et al., 2003). Observing an expression of disgust from an olfactory stimulus activates some of the same insular regions as experiencing personal disgust from an olfactory stimulus. These overlapping regions are in the left anterior insula and transitional regions between the insula and the left inferior frontal gyrus. In addition, similar regions of overlap were found in the right anterior cingulate cortex (Koukolik, 2012). The simulation of disgust in a social context and the idea of disgust activate the same neuronal network according to studies (Wicker et al., 2003).

Using the Terminology of Moral Emotions in Ordinary Language

Valerie Curtis referred to her research at local school, where teenagers said what is morally disgusting for them: "mocking someone in a crowd, bullying, racism, discrimination, standing by when other suffer, cloning babies, drug taking, suicide, bigotry, taking the Lord's name in vain, soldier deserting, spitting in someone face, government allowing injustice, putting profit before human life, exploitation of the poor, invading privacy, hypocrisy, back-stabbing a friend, poor sportsmanship, swearing, smoking when pregnant, vandalism, rape, adultery, treachery, stealing from the poor or handicapped, terrorism, chemical weapons, child slavery, cruelty to animals, pedophilia, incest, pornography, torture, wife beating, sadism, mistreatment of the elderly and vulnerable, cannibalism, eating dogs, murder, pollution" (Curtis, 2013, p. 77). In the academic year 2023–2024, I did a similar research with full-time and part-time students at The Faculty of Law, Comenius University in Bratislava. I received 97 answers from students aged 19 to 51 years: 61 respondents were women, 35 respondents were men, and 1 respondent claimed a different gender in the questionnaire. The first question was focused on respondents' associations with the term "disgust". The question literally read: List 10 words that you associate with the concept of disgust. Respondents most often mentioned expressions: loathing, revulsion, dislike, smell, toxicity, retching, nausea, violence, unwillingness, evil, compulsion, force, hatred, despite, resistance, against the will, fatigue, hopelessness, difficulties, failure, discord, discouragement, discomfort, rape, government, Slovakia, elections, lies, pedophilia, violence, botox, snake, poisoning, impossibility, trouble, annoying, negative, fatigue, apathy, stereotype, monotony, getting up, boredom, stress, time constraints, lack of motivation, restlessness, bad mood, disappointment, frustration. The second question was: List the mentioned concepts related to the word "disgust" in the order of their relevance (from the most relevant to the least relevant), and respondents answered most often: resistance, fatigue, loathing, revulsion, dislike, smell, nausea, hopelessness, difficulty, failure, disharmony, discouragement, discouragement, annoyance, snake, violence, rape. In the third question, I asked respondents about 10 words that they associate with the opposite of disgust. They answered: attraction, goodness, taste, will, love, sympathy, pleasant, fun, joy, willingness, fulfillment, meaning, pleasure, positivity, simplicity, fun, unpretentiousness, purposefulness, travelling, discovery, home, child, work, sun, rest, honesty, dialogue, nice, aesthetic, positive, clear, soup, adorable, light, warm, ambition, excitement, positivity, enthusiasm, curiosity, creativity, perseverance, willingness, enthusiasm, growth, overcoming, absence of fear, help. In the following question, the respondents had to list the mentioned opposites in the order of their relevance (from the most relevant to the least relevant). They answered mostly: joy, fulfillment, meaning, pleasure, positivity, simplicity, fun, unpretentiousness, purposefulness, enthusiasm, ambition, excitement, admiration, creativity, pleasantness, enchantment, wonder, comfort, satisfaction, relaxation, fragrance, beauty, relaxation. In the following question, the students were asked to state (specify) what disgusts them in public space (objects, situations, persons, etc.). They could list any number of objects that disgust them. They answered: feces, vomit, garbage, poorly sprayed buildings and premises, saliva, smell, unidentifiable liquids, vulgar, noisy people, dirty people, neglected people, neglected premises, political situation, injustice, disrespect, indifference, inconsideration, disorder, malice, unwillingness, objects on the sidewalks (waste bins, e-bikes, etc.), garbage, spit on the ground, starlings politics, coalition, ignoration, negative thinking people, alibism, stereotype, people's self-centeredness, lack of awareness of the environment as well as other people, bad use of public funds, people's behavior toward people serving other people (integrated rescue system). The next question was: Give reasons why the above objects in public space disgust you. (You can give any number of reasons.) Respondents answered mostly: they seem toxic, I'm afraid of contamination, I'm afraid that I'll catch viruses, bacteria, that I'll gag, that the smell/dirt will stick to me, poor standard of living, mood in society and I think the words themselves are self-explanatory. They disgust me as much as I am disgusted by the overall direction of a society that cannot exist as a whole, as everyone looks at the world only through their own perspective without regard for the perspective of others.

They are disgusting because politicians are conceited and think that they are God and can do everything, A negative thinking person transfers his mood to another. Alibism disgusts me because it demotivates and does not lead to solving the problem. People's complacency has grown to enormous proportions, and everyone only decides what is good for them not for society as such. The penultimate question was: State (specify) what disgusts you in natural space (objects, situations, persons, etc.). You can list any number of objects that evoke you. The most frequent answers were: garbage, decaying animal carcasses, worms, barriers, I am particularly disgusted by disrespect for nature, and I am most disgusted if I have known a natural place in Bratislava since birth (park, forest...) and it is destroyed for the purpose of building buildings. If I see something like this, I want to cry. Garbage, people, snakes, mess, lots of people, disrespect for nature as such. And the last question of the questionnaire was: Justify why the above-mentioned objects in public space disgust you. (You can give any number of reasons.) Respondents stated most often: garbage evokes the stupidity of people, I fear that it contaminates the environment, dead animals are disgusting because I'm afraid of bacteria, the sight of blood, internal organs and fluids limitation in space, because I think it is a basic duty of people to nature, to treat it with respect and to try to give back what it has given us, they have no purpose there because I'm afraid of them and they look disgusting, of course, garbage does not belong in the natural environment and everyone should respect that. Seeing garbage in nature dishonors the entire environment and nature itself. Natural monuments or places in nature that are too sought after by people lose their charm, and we don't enjoy them as much when there is a large mass of tourists around.

When we look at the terms that the respondents associate with the term "disgust", it is interesting that they associate not only physical manifestations or feelings that disgust them (odor, vomiting, spit, poison, botox, etc.) but also manifestations connected with immorality or social unacceptable behavior or actions (pedophilia, vulgarity, untruthfulness, lies, bad mood, frustration, hate, etc.) even with criminal acts (according to the Slovak Criminal Code No. 300/2005 Coll.), for example, rape or violence. Respondents also mentioned one animal, snake (surprisingly, spider was not mentioned in the questionnaire, although, in many researches, it is mentioned in connection with the experience of fear and disgust, i.e. Woody et al., 2005; Frynta et al., 2021; Çavusoglu & Dirik, 2011) and – (again surprisingly) feeling of stereotype, monotony, boredom, which are not often mention in literature in relation to the emotion of disgust. Student responses regarding the opposite of disgust are also interesting. The predominant answers were joy, fulfillment, or warmth, but they also considered the opposite of disgust specific meal (soup) or a feeling of warmth, a child, travel, i.e. all situations, feelings, and associations that are pleasant to specific subjects. Admiration as an opposite of disgust was mentioned by several respondents, but to a lesser extent than we expected. Respondents also reflected the emotions of disgust in the town, and they are disgusted by garbage, graffitied, and sprayed buildings, contaminated garbage cans, spit, dirty sidewalks, the lack of greenery, and the like. Let's look at approaches to the city and its own "emotionality" in philosophy.

Experiencing Emotions in Public Space (Especially in the City)

As Marcelli notes (Marcelli, 2011), the city is created in opposition to wild nature but gradually makes it its domestic (and necessary) part. Even Claude Lévi-Strauss comments: "...And the city, where nature and the human mind meet, is perhaps an even more precious reality than works of art." As a group of animals that enclose their biological history within its boundaries and at the same time as thinking beings model it with conscious intentions, the city, with its genesis and its form, is a stelae of the regularity of biological reproduction, organic development, and artistic creation. It is at the same time a natural object and a cultural subject, an individual and persons, a lived reality and a dreamed reality: it is a supremely human thing" (Lévi-Strauss 1966, p. 83). The greatest transformation of our ancestors began with tilling the land. "Tilling the land is already something, to an artificial, distant hunter and gatherer, it is a transformation of nature", as Osvald Spengler expressed it, "to cultivate does not mean to take something, but to produce" (Spengler, 2011, 392). Cultivating the soil becomes a prerequisite for the emergence of culture and even the city. All great cultures are urban. Spengler goes so far as to claim that world history is the history of urban people, which can be understood as saying that all religions, art, science, and political systems rest on one primitive phenomenon of humanity, the existence of the city (Spengler, 2011). It is a reasoning with which one can easily agree because, after all, everything that culture brings in religion, art, and leadership originated in cities. The peoples of the early cultures were gradually transformed into urban peoples. We know specifically the Indian or Chinese image of the city; we also talk about the specific English, Italian, German physiognomy of the city, and its related identity. What exactly is a city? A city is a public meeting space, a place where people come together to share their understanding of the world (Norberg-Schulz, 2015). As a gathering place of the public world, the city becomes an area of possibilities; we decide how, where, with whom to spend time, our identity develops here. "If we say that 'I am a New Yorker', it also means that the city also gives us a common identity (without us being the same as the other)" (Norberg-Schulz, 2015, p. 75). We do not have to use the offered possibilities of the city's public space; it is enough that we know about their existence, about their availability, in case of need. However, if a city loses its identity (e.g., by turning a city into a city), its population loses it too, and the identification "I'm a New Yorker" simply no longer applies. Identity is closely related to emotionality, we identify with cities, places, and objects through experiencing the emotions they evoke in us. For example, any building in the city represents, according to Norberg-Schulz (Norberg-Schulz, 2010), the so-called inhabited country, the space in which human life takes place. This space makes itself known as a mood, attunement, Norberg-Schulz uses the term "Stimmung" (Norberg-Schulz, 2015). He can be disgusted (by the smell, ugliness, dirt), he can feel anger (the facade of his favorite building has been changed or even demolished), horror, or sadness (the Notre Damme cathedral fire in Paris, in 2019), and so on. Emotionality, feelings, moods, atmosphere, "Stimmung" is ... obviously something intangible, and it is necessary to capture and embody it. This is done through buildings that reveal the properties of topography, material, vegetation, climate and light" (Norberg-Schulz, 2015, p. 90). Schulz recalls the role of identity that a healthy city should fulfill (Norberg-Schulz, 2015). Its role is not only to provide some primary pleasures but also to facilitate identification. So it should be a space that we easily identify with. The importance of experiencing emotionality in public space is an interesting contribution by the English Victorian theoretician of the cultural values of medieval architecture, August Welby Northmore Pugin. Pugin compared London in the past, embodied in Gothic architecture, and in the present, and he called his work from 1836 Contrasts, or a comparison of the noble buildings of the 14th and 15th centuries with similar buildings in our days showing the decay of taste, so we already perceive in the title his condemnation of the decaying present. He documents this phenomenon in a pair of paintings, where on one side he built medieval London, lofty Gothic churches, chapels, beautiful palaces, and on the other side their present parallels (Marcelli, 2011). He was later followed up and directly responded to by John Ruskin, who, during a lecture in Edinburgh, showed the audience a picture of a simple rectangular window made of massive blocks of stone and asked how many such windows they thought there were in Edinburgh's New Town, and then added that only in the morning in Queen Street he counted 678 plain windows without any ornament. With this, according to Marcelli (Marcelli, 2011), he wanted to support his initial thesis: "No mortal has ever been interested in such architecture as is being built at the present time, nor could it be interested" (Ruskin, 1853, p. 3). According to Ruskin, contemporary architecture is directed toward simplicity and does not arouse any aesthetic interest, any aesthetic emotion.

You can't admire her. Nor does it evoke disgust, wonder, sadness, or anger. It is impossible to identify with her. Let's move to the same time, i.e. in 1853 from Edinburgh to Paris where George Eugene Haussmann takes on the task of rebuilding the capital. Its goal is a rationally organized space in which the dynamism of big city movements will manifest itself. Where previously the dark streets of the medieval city center meandered, Haussmann opened wide boulevards to the flow of people, goods, and light. Interestingly, the motive for his actions was not the desire to free the masses of people from the unhealthy and dirty environment of the slums; he just wanted to free them from the grip of past centuries. He managed to transform the rotting and dirty center of Paris into a modern airy metropolitan environment. He created a sewage network, provided clean water supplies, and had parks and gardens built (Marcelli, 2011). His Paris evoked admiration, not disgust of the past. The expression of the connection of emotionality and the identification of an individual with parts of the public space of the city can also be found in the mythical Utopia by Thomas More, where the main character addresses words to the modern city (probably London): "There are also pubs, dens, a brothel on a brothel, wine bars, cellars, finally so many indecent games, dice on a board and in a funnel, cards, a ball, a ball, a disk" (More, 1978, p. 38). Clearly from Mor's description, we feel that the changes in public space that modern-day cities went through arouse emotions of disgust, indignation, and contempt. However, in the descriptions of Thomas More, we can find, among other things, the connection, interweaving of nature, biological and geographical aspects, and man, which I referred to right at the beginning of this text. The sea emphasizes that the coast of the mythical island is securely fortified, both by nature and by buildings, i.e. human creations. There are 54 cities on the island; the author describes them as well-built, spacious, all "...are as one, if the landscape allows it" (More, 1978, p. 51). And further, the author's reminder of the importance of connecting nature and the results of creative activities of man: "The streets are twenty feet wide, and behind all the houses are large orchards. They are surrounded by residential houses, which have an entrance from the street and an exit to the garden from the back... They take good care of their gardens, grow vines, fruits, herbs and flowers. Everything is so thoroughly laid out in them that I have never seen gardens as fruitful and beautiful as theirs" (More 1978, pp. 52-53).

Emotion of Admiration in More Detail

Admiration is an other-focused emotion (Ortony et al., 2011) elicited by virtue or skill above standards (Immordino-Yang, et al., 2009). Admiration belongs to positive emotions in response to an outstanding person or object. This emotion should serve to keep a person's ideals and values accessible as guides for behavior and also contribute to the adoption and internalization of ideals, values, and goals (Schindler et al., 2012). As mentioned in Schindler, "...admiration is elicited by outstanding role models who represent specific ideals or values. The excellence of such models, at least in principle, can be understood, matched, and even surpassed by others" (Schindler et al., 2012, p. 85–118). Moral function of admiration may be seen in encouraging others who aspire to grow by showing that it is possible to actualize ideals. The action tendencies associated with admiration are to uphold and honor ideals. The admiring one seeks to praise and affiliate with the other as well as to emulate the other's conduct. The primary function of admiration is to enhance the individual's agency in striving for ideals (Schindler et al., 2012). Etymology the word "admiration" is in English the noun of the verb admire, which is defined as "regard with respect or warm approval; look at with pleasure" (Compact Oxford Dictionary, 2003, p. 13). Etymology of the word "admiration" reaches into the early 15th century, from Old French admiration which means "astonishment, surprise" and from Latin admirationem "a wondering at, admiration", noun of state from past-participle stem of admirari "regard with wonder, be astonished", from ad "to; with regard to" and mirari "to wonder", from mirus which may be translated as "wonderful" .The sense has gradually weakened since 16th century toward "high regard, esteem". The Latin used term "admiratio", while we translate the prefix ad as "to" "onwards something" miró as "to look", so admiratio was used in the sense of wondering, being amazed, in awe. The Latin admiratio in the meaning of amazement or astonishment gradually weakened from the 16th century and took on the meaning of "to hold in respect". Admiration is one of the positive emotions, it is a present and expressed appreciation of someone or something, it is related to other positive emotions such as wonder, awe, adoration, fascination. According to Paul Ekman (Ekman, 2015), if we admire someone because he inspires us, for example, he arouses in us feelings similar to wonder. However, it is a separate emotion and must be distinguished from wonder. When experiencing the emotion of admiration, the same physiological changes do not occur as in the case of amazement; in the case of admiration, the accompanying physiological changes are the so-called goosebumps, changes in breathing, possibly shaking the head (Ekman, 2015). "We want to follow the object of our admiration, we feel drawn to it, but in amazement we just stand still, we have no need for any action" (Ekman, 2015, p. 328). For example in Slovak language admiration is translated as obdiv. The etymology of this term refers to the expression to look. The expression to look, used in Proto-Slavic since the 15th century (divati se), derives from the Indo-European "dei-" which can be translated as "to shine", "to shine", "to shine". The connection can also be seen with the words "theater" (in the older sense, the term "theater" meant an illustrative example, a model, what someone is looking at), "spectator". From the term "to look" came "to admire" and "to wonder". However, the etymology of the term "admiration" also refers to the expression to wonder. The derivations are then astonishment, wondering, wondrous, strangely (Králik, 2015). Diana Onu, Thomas Kessler, and Joanne Smith made systematical conception of admiration, where one of the most interesting aspects of this emotion is, what it does, the kind of behaviors it facilitates. They discuss the consequences of admiration as they occur at the intraindividual level (consequences for the admirer), interpersonal level or inter group level for group-based admiration (consequences for the relationship), and group and cultural level (consequences for the group) (Onu et al., 2016). Onu et al. referred to Haidt (2009) who also found specific relationship consequences following admiration; participants who felt admiration reported intentions to enhance the reputation of the admired target by praising them to others, and to acknowledge their performance (Haidt, 2009; Onu et al., 2016). Onu and colleagues found evidence that group-based admiration is associated with willingness to receive help from an admired outgroup. In a study on national group members eactions to more successful countries, they found that admiration for a high-performing outgroup is related only to a desire for autonomy-related help (e.g., receiving training or guidance to improve) from a higher-status outgroup but not dependency-oriented help (e.g., donations). Emotion of admiration characterizes how people feel toward those they see as allies and with whom they wish to cooperate (as I will show bellow, in the section on leader and authority). Henrich and Gil-White considered admiration as a unique cultural transmission factor in human groups: "[A]dmiration makes it easier for skilled group members to approach and acquire skills from them, thereby facilitating the spread of superior skills within the group. These admired individuals are also praised for their skill, increasing their prestige within the group" (Henrich and Gil-White, 2001, p. 176). Henrich and Gil-White suggest that the admiration of subordinates toward superiors characterizes a certain type of social hierarchy, which is based on acquired prestige (Henrich & Gil-White, 2001). Sweetman et al. (2013) tested the effect of admiration on social hierarchy and found that admiration for higher-status members promotes hierarchy maintenance. In connection with the emotion of admiration, it is interesting that we also experience it toward persons (or situations, characteristics, events, etc.) that we would not evaluate as moral or exemplary worthy of imitation. We admire politicians, celebrities, people from show business, etc. many times not because of their moral qualities but because of the charm of their personality or various talents (sometimes even the talent to lie, mislead, speak angrily, create an enemy, etc., persons like Hitler, Stalin, Goebbels, Heydrich, Mussolini, and many others are admired by some individuals or social groups decades and even centuries after their death despite immoral influence).

Much of what we like and admire can be classified as kitsch. In search of the roots of attraction, Milan Kundera thought of modern culture as important sources of kitsch: "[T]he aesthetics of the mass media necessarily become the aesthetics of kitsch and how mass media penetrate more and more into our lives, kitsch becomes aesthetic and moral code" (Kundera, 1985, p. 13). In his novel The Unbearable Lightness of Being, the term "kitsch" becomes the center of the author's reflections, although he hesitated to use it according to his own words (Kundera, 1988, p. 64), as the term was almost unknown in French at the time or used only in an impoverished sense. Kundera pointed out that in the translations of Hermann Broch into French, the translators of his Kitsch reached for a translation "art de pacotille", "junk ar", i.e. "junk art" (Kundera, 1988, p. 64). And kitsch represents much more than just worthless, low-quality art; there is a kitsch attitude, kitsch behavior, just a "kitsch need for kitsch" (Kundera, 1988, p. 64). Kundera further sees it as a human need to look into the mirror of a beautifying lie and let yourself be moved to tears breastfeeding during self-reflection (Kundera, 1988). Tomáš Kulka pointed out that there is no agreement among etymologists regarding the origin of the term: "[S]omeone believe that the word 'kitsch' originated from the English term "sketch") garbled by German pronunciation. Ludwig Giesz comes to mind, that 'kitsch' is derived from the verb 'kitschen', which means 'day of Strasssenschlam zusammenscharren' – something like scooping up mud from the street. There exists also conjectures that 'kitsch' was created by the inversion of the French term 'chic'. However, experts agree that since its birth in the second half of the 19th century, this term has clear negative connotations" (Kulka, 2014, p. 33). Even so, we like kitsch objects, situations, and attitudes; we seek them out, they move us, and we cry next to them. Emberto Eco also analyzed the emotionality of kitsch; according to him, the main feature of kitsch is the effort to achieve an effect in the area feelings, to offer a ready-made, annotated emotion ready for use and feeling. Objective content is then not nearly as important as impression, effect, or emotion. For example, literary kitsch understands eco as artisticIa lie. Its goal is not to drag the reader to active knowledge, research, and reflecting but forcing him to submit to the effect just to survive the effect here alone, in the illusion that it is precisely in this emotional experience that he lies under state of experience with beauty (Eco, 1995). Robert Solomon, on the other hand, advocates the phenomenon of kitsch, and critics' opposition to it stems from an unwillingness to tolerate any kind of emotion that is considered too sentimental or "sweet". Solomon argues that this attack on sentimentalism is in fact it attacks emotions themselves and opposes emotionless coldness and cynicism (Solomon, 1991). However, this Solomon insight seems a little disparaging, if we consider the studies on the relationship between kitsch and politics, primarily totalitarian. Apart from Kundera's exposure of kitsch as the main tool for mass control in a communist society, it is interesting to probe the analysis of Saul Friedlander, who showed the role of kitsch in the mobilization of the masses in Hitler's Germany (Friedlander, 1986). Kitsch can become a truly dangerous phenomenon if the masses are seduced by it. Mass man is not subject to rationality, but to impulse. Another characteristic feature of the mass is the simplification of feelings. The causes of the crowd man were analyzed by Ortega Y Gasset in the book Revolt of the Crowds, and he sees them in the accumulation factor of "fullness": "...cities are full of people. Houses full of tenants. Hotels full of guests. Trains full of passengers. Cafes full of visitors. Streets full of pedestrians. The waiting rooms of the best doctors are full of patients. Theaters, if they are not too out of date, full of spectators...What was not a problem before becomes almost permanent: to find a place" (Gasset, 1993). The key is an admiring, sentimental, cheesy attitude toward the main idea that unites the masses or toward the leader they look up to. In the mass, all individual faculties are lost, and the actions of each member are directed in one direction, to a common goal. In the crowd, educated people with above-average intelligence meet people whose cognitive abilities are limited. According to the psychologist Le Bon, who was one of the first to study the psychology of the crowd, the crowd is not capable of producing actions that require higher intelligence and recognition of the lure of kitsch (Le Bon, 2016). Mass society creates a space for the presentation of the weak; that is why, it is so attractive. An individual in a crowd gains confidence that he is part of a larger number of people, that he lives for a common idea, a goal he admires. In the mass, the individual is anonymous, so he easily loses his sense of responsibility and allows himself to be carried away by impulsive actions. Every idea or action that appears in the crowd is contagious, impression spreads quickly, and suggestibility, i.e. susceptibility, to accepting other people's ideas is another characteristic of a mass person. Another characteristic feature of the mass is the simplification of feelings. This means that mixed feelings, uncertainty, or doubts about the main idea of the crowd or the leader have no place here. Since the mass is always oriented in one direction, it does not create space for discussion, resistance, and disagreement. According to Arendt, the masses were born out of a highly atomized society where the rivalry structure and associated loneliness of the individual was mitigated by party membership and admiration to party and its ideas. Only a strong individual who can act as an authority earns the admiration and sympathy of the crowd. One of the typical characteristics of groupthink is the presence of a strong authority. We attribute the position of leader to a person who stands above the mass of people. As Arendt states, his place is at the center of the movement and represents not only the source but also the driving force of the movement. The leader is the one who influences the crowd and asserts his authoritative position. He is the bearer of propaganda through which he becomes a functionary of the controlled masses. At the same time, the crowd is a herd that cannot do without a master for whom it feels the emotion of admiration (Le Bon, 2016). The leader becomes an admired hero, whom the crowd applauds and recognizes without limit. If we disrespected him, mocked him, or felt disgusted with him, he would never become a leader.

Conclusion

We have come to the end of the text, which begins with the imaginary color of emotions and ends with the phenomenon of the leader. I tried to show the various shades of the emotion of admiration and disgust, which I considered to be opposites in several previous texts. In this text, I showed more colorful synonyms and opposites of the moral emotions of disgust and admiration (the opposite of disgust can be, for example, the emotion of joy, a feeling of warmth). I also tried to show the differences in the meaning of the terms "emotions", "feelings", and "affects". The morally and socially most important impact of the emotion of admiration I find is in uncritical admiration, which leads to fanatical or ideological worship of authority or leader. Such an experience of admiration gradually leads to the destruction of communities, as history has shown many times.

References

Aristotle. (2009). *The Nicomachean Ethics.* Oxford University Press.

Aristotle. (2013). *The Art of Rhetoric.* Harper Collins.

Cambridge International Dictionary of English. (1995). Procter, P. (ed.) Cambridge University Press.

Compact Oxford Dictionary (2003). Oxford University Press.

Curtis, V. (2013). *Don´t Look, Don´t Touch, Don´t Eat.* University of Chicago Press.

Damasio, A. R. (1994). *Descartes´s Error.* New York: Avon Books.

Damasio, A. R. (2000). *The Feeling of What Happens: Body and Emotion in the Making of Consciousness.* Mariner Books.

Darwin, Ch. (2020). *Výraz emocí u člověka a u zvířat.* [The Expression of the Emotions in Man and Animals] Portál.

Démuth, A. (2019). *Beauty, Aesthetic Experience, and Emotional Affective States.* Peter Lang.

Descartes, R. (1989). *The Passions of the Soul.* Hackett Publishing.

Eco, U. (1995). *Skeptikové a tešitelé,* [Apocalittici e integrati] Nakladatelství svoboda.

Ekman, P. (2009). Darwin's Contributions to Our Understanding of Emotional Expressions. *Philosophical Transactions of the Royal Society B: Biological Sciences. 364*(1535), 3449–3451.

Ekman, P. (2015). *Emotion in the Human Face.* Malor Books.

Ekman P., Friesen W. V. & Ellsworth P. (1972). *Emotion in the Human Face: Guidelines for Research and an Integration of Findings.* Pergamon Press

Franco, A. B. (2006). *Descartes Theory of Passions.* University of Pittsburgh.

Friedlander, S. (1986). *Reflections of Nazism: An Essay on Kitsch and Death.* Avon Books.

Frijda, N. H. (1986). *The Emotions.* Cambridge University Press.

Gasset, Y. O. (1993). *Vzpoura davů.* [La rebelion de las masas] Naše vojsko.

Gray, J. A., & McNaughton, L. (2003). *The Neuropsychology of Anxiety: An Enquiry into the Functions of the Septo-Hippocampal System.* Oxford University Press.

Haidt, J. (2003). *Moral Emotions,* Oxford University Press.

Haidt, J. (2013): *The Righteous Mind.* Penguin Books.

Hofmann, W., Kotabe, H. P., Vohs, K. D., & Baumeister, R. F. (2015). Desire and desire regulation. In W. Hofmann & L. F. Nordgren (eds.), *The Psychology of Desire.* New York: Guilford, 61–81.

Kišoňová, R. (2021). The social emotions of disgust and admiration in the context of language. *Language, Individual and Society, 15,* 22–27.

Kišoňová, R. (2022). A Few Remarks towards Environmental Aesthetics. Aesthetics of Landscapes and Its Impact on Human Emotions. *Studia Ecologiae et Bioethicae*, 20(4), 1–11. doi.org/10.21697/seb.2022.18

Kišoňová, R. (2023). Considering the emotion of disgust in the context of terminology and contemporary literature. In A. Démuth, S. Démuthová (eds.), *A Conceptual and Semantic Analysis of the Qualitative Domains of Aesthetic and Moral Emotions: An Introduction*. Peter Lang, 81–100.

Koukolík, F. (2012). *Lidský mozek*. [Human Brain] Galén.

Králik, L. (2015). *Stručný etymologický slovník slovenčiny*. [A Concise Etymological Dictionary of Slovak] Veda.

Kulka, T. (2014). *Umění a kýč*. [Art and kitsch] Torst.

Kundera, M. (1985). Man Thinks, God Laughs. *New York Review*, 13(6) 11–12.

Kundera, M. (1988). *The Art of the Novel*. The Grove Press.

Le Bon, G. (2016). *Psychologie davu*. [The Crowd: A Study of the Popular Mind] Portál.

Lee, K.H., & Siegel, G. J. (2009). Common and Distinct Brain Networks Underlying Explicit Emotional Evaluation: A Meta-analytic Study. *Social Cognition Affect Neuroscience*, 10, https://doi.org/10.1093/scan/nsp001.

Lévi-Strauss, C. (1966). *Smutné tropy*. [Tristes Tropiques] Odeon.

Marcelli, M. (2011). *Mesto vo filozofii*. [City in Philosophy] Kalligram.

More, T. (1978). *Utopie*. [Utopia] Mladá fronta.

Norberg-Schulz, Ch. (2015). *Principy moderní architektury*. [Principles of Modern Architecture] Malvern.

Onu, D., Kessler, T., & Smith, J. R. (2016). Admiration: A Conceptual Review. *Emotion Review*, 8(3), 218–230. https://doi.org/10.1177/1754073915610438.

Ortony, A., Clore, G., L., & Collins, A. (2011). *The Cognitive Structure of Emotions*. Cambridge University Press. https://doi.org/10.1017/CBO9780511571299

Pessoa, L. (2013). *The Cognitive-Emotional Brain: From Interactions to Integration*. Oxford University Press.

Prasanthi, J., & Prakash, K. N. (2020). *Human Emotion Recognition from Face Images: Recognition and Retrieval of Emotions from Facial Expression*. LAP Lambert Academic Publishing.

Ruskin, J. (1853). *Lectures on Architecture and Painting. Delivered at Edinburgh in November 1853*. John Wiley.

Shweder, R. A. (1994). "You're not sick, you're just in love": Emotion as an interpretive system. In Ekman P., Davidson R. J. (eds.), *The Nature of Emotion: Fundamental Questions*. New York, NY: Oxford University Press, 32–44.

Schindler, I., Zink, V., Menninghaus, W. et al. (2012). Admiration and Adoration: Their Different Ways of Showing and Shaping Who We Are. *Cognition & Emotion*, 27(1).

Simon, M. (2003). *Facial Expressions*. Watson-Guptill Publications,

Solomon, R. C. (1991). On Kitsch and Sentimentality, *The Journal of Aesthetics and Art Criticism*, *49* (1) 1–14.

Spengler, O. (2011). *Zánik Západu*. [Der Untergang des Abendlandes. Umriss einer Morphologie der Weltgeschichte]. Academia.

Helen, M., McColl, A., Damasio, H., & Damasio, A. (2009). Neural Correlates of Admiration and Compassion. *Proceedings of the National Academy of Sciences*, *106*(19), 8021–8026. https://doi.org/10.1073/pnas.0810363106

Wicker B., Keysers, Ch., Plailly J., Royet, J. P., & Gallese, V. G. (2003). Both of Us Disgusted in My Insula: The Common Neural Basis of Seeing and Feeling Disgust. *Neuron 40*(3), 655–664. doi 10.1016/s0896-6273(03)00679-2.

Anger
The Awareness of Evil and the Defiant Decision to Take Justice into One's Own Hands

Andrej Démuth

> *Showing your emotions is like a bleeding next to a shark.*
>
> English proverb

Introduction

Anger is one of the most pronounced and perhaps the most common human feelings or emotions. Some consider it to be a basic emotion (e.g., Ekman 1999) from which many other feelings or emotions are derived (e.g., a child's first cry can be seen as an expression or derivative of some form of anger). Others – beginning with Descartes (Descartes, 1649/2002) – believe that anger is a secondary emotion that is derived from other more basic states and feelings (e.g., resentment and hatred). Here anger appears as a reaction to other feelings and states that are taking place in our bodies or our environment (especially pain, fear, frustration...). According to Damasio (Damasio, 1999), while primary emotions are mostly innate complex reactions of the body to some stimuli (they are automatically triggered by them), secondary emotions can be understood as the body's somatic response to these states and thus they are an expression of how we feel when we feel something. It is not the object of this chapter to contribute to the age-old war over the existence, nature, and exhaustive definition of these basic emotions, or whether anger is one of them. Rather, we wish to focus the attention of the reader on the definition of the problem – what is anger, what we mean by it, and everything that is associated with it by the one who feels it, as well as what is in the mind of the one who speaks of it. Anger, like many other emotions, does not represent a feeling or phenomenon that is quite clear and uncontaminated. On the contrary, very often it is associated with many other feelings that mark it and influence its perception. Therefore, pure anger is not experienced as easily as it may seem at first sight; this further muddies the possibility that we have a correct and deep understanding of it. As with other feelings, our language does not have an adequate number of terms that can be used to clearly distinguish the subtle distinctions between different feelings, and it is often the case that we are unable to precisely express the different shades of meaning involved in a given mental state, which in turn can (and often does) lead to misunderstandings when we try to communicate them.

As Riccardo Williams states, "anger is probably one of the mostly debated basic emotions, owing to difficulties in detecting its appearance during development, its functional and affective meaning (is it a positive or a negative emotion?), especially in human beings. Behaviors accompanied by anger and rage serve many different purposes and the nuances of aggressive behaviors are often defined by the symbolic and cultural framework and social contexts. Nonetheless, recent advances in neuroscientific and developmental research, as well as clinical psychodynamic investigation, afford a new view on the role of anger in informing and guiding many aspects of human conducts" (Williams, 2017).

One such new view may be the attempt to apply the geometry of thinking (feeling) to the mapping and experience of individual emotions.

The geometry of thinking is a philosophical concept from the philosopher Peter Gärdenfors (Gärdenfors, 2000). It is a cognitive theory of semantics that proposes that the meanings of words can be described in terms of geometric structures. Concepts are a kind of semantic points or spaces that are defined by the basic semantic dimensions that describe the individual features of the concepts in question. Through the different saturations of the same or adjacent dimensions, the individual meanings of concepts can then be compared. An example of this way of thinking is the description of individual colors through their color, saturation and intensity. Each color represents a convex region in a given color space that can be grasped by a similar convex semantic region – a concept. Concepts then delineate the given natural convex regions by defining their boundaries. Importantly, the convexity of the given regions allows us to interpret their foci as prototypes of categories. That is, any hue of the same color (e.g., yellow) is closer to a prototype of that color than to any other color. Gärdenfors used this strategy to describe the semantic content of individual concepts, where all possible shades of yellow fall within the convex conceptual space belonging to the concept yellow.

A similar strategy to Gärdenfors has been used by several researchers to map basic mental states. Fushun Wang and Alfredo Perera Jr. (Wang, Pereira, 2016), for example, believe that all emotional states can be explained using a geometric spatial model whose main qualitative dimensions (axes) represent the various neuromodulators involved in their production. They identified dopamine, which is responsible for pleasant feelings, serotonin, which appears with unpleasant feelings and disgust, norepinephrine, which is characteristic of feelings associated with surprise and activity (this includes, e.g., fear, but also anger and aggression), and finally, the fourth axis is represented by acetylcholine. The latter appears in relatively calm emotional states such as contentment and anticipation. Wang and Pereira thus present a model of the geometry of feelings and emotional states that makes it possible to describe any emotional state in an imaginary space formed by the basic neuromodulators and their associated qualities of feeling. Each feeling is then represented by a geometric point in that space whose location can be described through the degree of saturation of each dimension. Anger in such a model inevitably represents a convex complex space whose main dimensions are increased activity (caused by noradrenaline) as an immediate response to some unwanted stimulus but also disgust (unpleasantness) or liking (pleasantness), depending on the amount of serotonin or dopamine secreted. The problem with Wang's concept is the assumption that emotions are only formed through the participation of individual isolated neuromodulators, rather than by their interaction. Wang and Pereira assumed that only pleasant feelings (dopamine) can be felt at a given time, without the participation of any unpleasant feelings (serotonin). Similarly, they view the action of noradrenaline and acetylcholine to be antagonistic. In reality, however, many feelings are produced by an interaction of all the neuromodulators and thus there are pleasant feelings of sadness and nostalgia, as well as pleasant, but also unpleasant, feelings of worry, etc. It even seems that most emotional states are of such a mixed nature, and pure, prototypical emotions are very rare.

The Question of the Opposite of Anger

Wang's concept assumes the existence of opposite feelings according to the degree of saturation of the individual neuromodulators. If anger is associated with norepinephrine, the opposite feeling should be that which is associated with its absence, or even antagonism. Thus, the first dimension could be the dimension of activity. In Wang's case, then, it should be something calm. Therefore, many think that a feeling of calm or patience is the opposite of immediate and impulsive anger.

However, Robert Plutchik (Plutchik, 1982), in his famous theory of emotion, posits that fear is the counterpart of anger. The reason for his reasoning is that while angry we are oriented toward the object that causes it, when we experience fear we run away from it. In this sense, fighting and being ready to fight is the opposite of an escape strategy. This is also recognized by Wang, who considers both feelings to involve a response associated with the secretion of norepinephrine, but differently in each case. So, it is not just about being activated but also about the vector (the direction) along which the activity is directed.

Both anger and fear share a rejection of what triggers them. Therefore, their opposites should rather be acceptance. Most of our respondents reported the feeling or emotion of love as the opposite of anger. This too is directed toward the object, but not for the purpose of removing it, but rather for the purpose of accepting it. Love, however, does not always have to be eager, but can also be calm – tolerant and respectful.

Another dimension of perception is a subjective reflection on the pleasantness or pleasure of the sensations experienced. In the case of anger, it is mostly an unpleasant feeling that is a reaction to something surprising. Its opposite, in the pleasantness dimension, is joy and pleasure. We get angry at that which does not please us and vice versa.

The Cambridge Dictionary lists the following opposites of anger: love, liking, fondness, good will, peacefulness, gentleness, amiability, approval, acceptance, condonation, calmness, equanimity, pleasure, gratification, forgiveness. Thus, it also notes the acceptance of what makes us angry, as we come to terms with it and do not want to change it through our own efforts. Either because we cannot (the opposite would then be apathy and resignation) or because we do not think it is appropriate – tolerance, forgiveness (Cambridge University Press, 2024).

From a deeper psychological-philosophical point of view, we might consider anger to be a manifestation of implicit self-confidence and a form of self-centeredness. Therefore, we allow ourselves to express it. If we are angry, we believe that it makes sense to express our anger – that it will make a difference. On the other hand, sometimes it is an expression of helplessness or powerlessness – why else would we express it if we could change the situation ourselves?

It seems, then, that anger has no single-unambiguous opposite and that in both the neuromodular and emotional or semantic planes, its opposites are different states of body and mind depending on which dimension – the plane of judgment – we are considering. For there is no anger like anger, and therefore its opposites are not identical either. All this encourages us to even more closely examine its nature and meanings.

The History of Anger and Its Exploration

As we have already mentioned, anger, according to several thinkers, is one of the basic emotions. It is not surprising, therefore, that in the history of European literature and Western culture-shaping writings, anger holds a prominent place as one of the first emotions to be mentioned and described on its own. For example, Homer's *Iliad*, the story of Achilles, is actually an epic of just and unjust anger; the first pages of the Bible, Genesis, where the first sin and divine anger in reaction to it are described, but also the first extra-ritual offense, Cain's murder of Abel as a consequence of anger for divine favor... (see Démuth, 2024), can be seen as such works. In the history of philosophy, anger was given attention as early as Plato, who thematized it in the dialogues, the *Republic*, the *Gorgias*, the *Euthyphro*, and the *Timaeus*. Aristotle explored it in a famous passage of his *Rhetoric*, where he presented it as one of the most complex and distinctive of human emotions, that has bodily, psychological, social, and moral dimensions. He viewed it as "a painful desire for revenge caused by a perceived undeserved slight", and thus as a desire for justice. The Stoic, Lucius Anaeus Seneca, considered anger to be such a significant and dangerous phenomenon that he devoted three books to it, entitled *De Irae*. Seneca was aware of the harmful effects of anger, not only in a social context but also within the personal life of an individual. Like Horatius (Horace, *Epistles*, 1. 2. 62), he regarded it as a brief madness ("Ira furor brevis est") - anger, as a bestial passion, in this vein anger was also addressed by his followers (e.g., Cicero, Plutarch) as well as thinkers throughout the Middle Ages and the modern period. In particular, we have learned to see anger as a loss of control, as an instability that limits our cognitive and volitional competence (anger as irrational/maladaptive), as a weakness or even a sin (insanity, sin, or demonic possession) when directed at another. Since the Renaissance, we have thematized the differences between the anger of men and women, of just and unjust anger, the anger of the gods, and the anger of man (Potegal, Novaco, 2010).

If we look into scholarly writings, for example, articles indexed in the *PubMed* database, we find that, as with other topoi, there has been a geometric increase in the number of works on anger. While the first articles on anger only began to appear in the database in 1945, even if only a few each year (1), in 2022 alone more than 3,200 articles were added to the database, and this rate has continued (Pubmed, 2024).

The most common topic associated with research into anger is anger management and coping theories. However, we also find investigations into the neural and neurobiological mechanisms of anger (Gilam and Hendler, 2017), its impact on the perception of information and misinformation (Greenstein and Franklin, 2020), risk assessments and risk-taking (Staicu and Cutov, 2010), and its relationship to empathy (Weblen et al., 2021), (in)justice (Miller et al., 2022), pain (Yarns, Cassidy, Jimenez, 2022), or intersex differences (Van Doren, Soto, 2021), among others. Alongside this, from time to time, there are also works with a more complex focus exploring the very nature of anger, its evolutionary role - both from the perspective of society and the individual, and from the perspective of cross-cultural differences. Examples of such works include the edited collection from Myisha Cherry and Owen Flanagan, published in 2017, that explores anger from a moral psychological perspective, or the work of a collective led by Agnes Callard in 2020, which summarized a wide-ranging discussion from The *Boston Review* featuring Paul Bloom, Jesse Prinz, Elisabeth Bruenig, Desmond Jagmohan, Victoria Spring and Daryl Cameron, Myisha Cherry, Rachel Achs, Barbara Herman, and Oded Na'aman, augmented by studies by Martha C. Nussbaum, Judith Butler, David Constan, Whitney Phillips, and Amy Olberding (all in: Callard 2020a). Equally paradigmatic was the book by Martha C. Nussbaum on anger and forgiveness (Nussbaum 2016) or, more recently, Owen Flanagan's, *How to Do Things with Emotions: The Morality of Anger and Shame across Cultures* (Flanagan 2021), which thematizes anger and its manifestations, including acceptance across cultures. Flanagan (like surprisingly argues) shows that anger is perceived differently at different times and in different cultures, not only in its means of expression but also in how it is evaluated and accepted. He argues that there are cultures that do not even have a separate word for anger, since it is almost non-existent, or that in some places it is associated with sadness and in others with pain. Flanagan points to the general prevalence and acceptability of anger in Western culture, whereas in some other cultural contexts anger is seen as a failure, a lack of nurture, control, and humility. For evolutionary reasons, Flanagan points to the epidemic nature of anger in a Western world shaped by liberal democracy and nurture, which (dis)corresponds with Dixon's understanding of anger as a modern contemporary concept. Dixon (Dixon, 2020) challenges the diagnosis of the present as an "age of anger", and with reference to the works of linguists and anthropologists, and ancient philosophical and literary texts, he explains that "anger" is a modern English word with no stable transhistorical reference. At the same time, therefore, he proposes the linguistic method as a way to avoid anachronisms and essentialism in the study of emotions (Dixon. 2020).

Anger in the Context of Related Concepts and Terms

In order to understand what we commonly mean by anger, it can be quite beneficial to look at the etymology and various synonyms or connotations of anger in different historical, social, and cultural contexts.

It has been shown that the ancient Greeks had thirteen different terms for anger and its various connotations or forms in Homer's writings alone. The basic Homeric Greek term for anger is Ménos. The *Iliad* that describes the Wrath of Achilles begins with this word. However, the Greek term "Ménos" does not mean anger as such. According to Leonard Muellner, "Menis means more than an individual's emotional response" (Muellner, 2005). On the basis of the epic exemplifications of the word, Muellner defines the term as "a cosmic sanction against behavior that violates the most basic rules of human society" (Muellner, 2005). However, the same Muellner, referring to Redfield, states that Ménis can be seen "as 'anger that is dangerous to someone', as anger seen from the outside" (Muellner, 2005). Thus, it is not a subjective feeling, but rather an expression, a revelation. Thus, it is a divine-righteous anger that can only be seen from the outside as a reaction to a violation of the rules.

The Greeks, however, also use other words for anger. The term "thumos" denotes the emotion in general. It is anger, passion, desire, or an inner urge, something that drives us from within. Thumós is derived from thyō, "to rush, to become hot, to breathe violently," and it is about passion-driven behavior, i.e., actions that arise from strong impulses (intense emotions). In people, it is an expression of passion, specifically the outburst and discharge of anger. At the same time, however, it is also something that resembles a spirit, living energy, that can be spoken to, that can be personified.

In contrast, the term "orgé" (from orgáō, "to become overwhelmed, puffed up, even constitutionally opposed") represents an intense anger, sometimes bordering on madness, that stems from an inner disposition in which we persistently oppose someone or something on the basis of our personal attitude.

Alongside this we have terms such as aganaktésis (indignation) communicating a sense of irritation, chalepaino (annoyance), kotos (resentment) which is characterized by duration, cholos (expressing bitterness, literally "bile"). Parorgismos is more about irritation and exasperation, σκύζεσθαι ((growl with anger), ménis – rage, or nemesis, which denotes a desire for revenge and retribution. Walsh points out that anger has such a strong cohort of synonyms in Greek that it raises the question of whether the above terms are really synonyms, or whether there is a fundamental difference in meaning between them that makes it impossible to grasp them all under a single central concept.

Similarly, in Slovak (Pisárčiková, 2004) we can find a number of concepts related to the word "anger": a feeling and expression of violent agitation ("rozčúlenie", "pobúrenie", referring to a storm ("búrka") of feelings and passions), indignation (rozhorčenie, indicating a state of bitterness in the body), but also anger ("zlosť", derived from malice or evil, "zlo"), poison ("jed", poisoning everything it comes into contact with), heart ("srd", referring to the place we experience anger, in our hearts ("srdce")), rage ("bes", similar to rabies), or bile ("žlč", indicating bitterness in the mouth). In a figurative sense, hatred is also synonymous with hate, with which it is often confused.

In English, we find synonyms such as annoyed, bitter, enraged, exasperated, furious, heated, impassioned, indignant, irate, irritable, irritated, mad, offended, outraged, resentful, sullen, uptight, affronted, antagonized, chafed, choleric, convulsed, cross, displeased, ferocious, fierce, fiery, fuming, galled, hateful, hot, huffy, ill-tempered, incensed, inflamed, infuriated, irascible, ireful, maddened, nettled, piqued, pissed, pissed off, provoked, put out, raging, riled, sore, splenetic, storming, sulky, vexed, wrathful, that refer to an unkind and irritable mood, unpleasant bitter tastes, irritability, fire and boiling blood, loss of control and discrimination, fierce fixation on the object of anger, burning, pain, and many other aspects.

Similarly, in German one can find many synonyms for the term "anger" (Wut) with some that cannot quite be translated into other languages (see the difference between Zorn and Wut – Oster, 2014).

Thus, the concept of anger seems to function as an umbrella concept that covers a number of distinct but semantically similar concepts and terms. In order to clarify meaning, different concepts convey their meaning in different ways and in doing so they also focus on quite different domains of meaning (taste, temperature, irritation, loss of control, hostility, etc.). In the following section, we will focus on the clarification of the concept of anger by distinguishing it from the concept of hatred, which is used as a similar term in many languages.

Anger and Hatred

Hatred, according to various definitions, is: (n.) a hostile emotion that combines intense feelings of detestation, anger, and often a desire to do harm – also called hatred (APA 2018). According to the *Penguin Dictionary of Psychology* it is: "a deep enduring, intense emotion expressing animosity, anger, and hostility toward a person, group or object. Hatred is usually assumed to be characterised by (a) the desire to harm or cause pain to the object of the emotion and (b) feelings of pleasure from the object's misfortunes" (Reber 1995, p. 330). It manifests (1) as a noun: "(a) intense hostility and aversion usually deriving from fear, anger, or sense of injury; (b) extreme dislike or disgust; (2) as a verb: (a) to feel extreme enmity toward; to regard with active hostility, (b) to have a strong aversion to; find very distasteful" (Merriam-Webster 2024).

In this context, hate is primarily defined as an emotion. In reality, however, it is an attitude rather than an emotion. Martin Heidegger, in his notes on Nietzsche's understanding of affectivity, distinguishes between anger and hatred, suggesting that hatred is a holistic attitude that reflects both a person's value orientation, cognitive beliefs, and their bodily experience of a given situation. Hate, according to Heidegger, is possible "only because it [hate] has already possessed us, only because it has grown in us for a long time, and, as we say, has been nourished in us" (Heidegger 1996, p. 45). Its roots, then, are deep. It did not arise all at once but is a result of the sedimentation of previous experiences (whether one's own or transferred from others). This is also why, if we hate, it is not just some minor aspect of something that bothers us. We hate "the whole existence of that which is the source of it.

What we are concerned with is the very being of the object hated. Therefore, everything associated with that object/person irritates us. In this respect, hatred is complex, and object-centred – focused on the very being of that which we hate – as well as in terms of residence – based on the very essence of our existence" (Démuth, 2024a, p. 97). We hate with our whole soul, and this manifests itself in our bodily manifestations. Hatred is constant and yet deep. It affects our minds and also our bodily functions much like anger (Démuth, 2024b).

However, unlike hatred, anger is primarily a feeling. Feelings are something that enable us to encounter an object. Psychologists think about feelings; in the most general way 1. "feeling refers to 'experiencing', 'sensing', or 'having a conscious process'. More specific meanings are: 2. Sensory impressions, which provide feelings from warmth to pain; 3. Affective states, as in a feeling of well-being, depression, desire etc.; 4. One of the dimensions of the emotion, particularly where the reference is on hypothesised elementary emotional continua such as Wundt's three dimensions of feelings; 5. Belief as in a vague feeling about something, not supported by any real evidence" (Reber 1995, p. 284). Feelings (German: das Gefühl) are thus mainly what we perceive; they enable us to feel the presence of both self and stimulus. They occur at receptors – at the interface between the subject and the active stimulus – and are actually an awareness of an encounter.

Antonio Damasio thinks of sensations as bodily markers, i.e., as an unconscious response to any internal or external stimulus which activates neural patterns in the brain. "It consists of having mental images arising from the neural patterns which represent the changes in body and brain that make up an emotion" (Damasio 1999, p. 280). So, a feeling of anger, is a more or less automatic response to stimuli that the organism encounters within its immediate environment, which it evaluates as socially or morally undesirable. This corresponds to Heidegger's understanding of feelings. Heidegger understands feelings as the openness of an organism to the action of something, which in turn fills us (füllen) with conscious experience – phenomena. However, anger is a little more complicated.

Anger as a Feeling or Emotion

Heidegger understands anger as an immediate reaction of an organism to an unwanted stimulus. In terms of Nietzsche's concept of affect as volition, it is a kind of automatic immediate response. The peculiarity of this reaction, however, is that on one hand it is the result of innate or learning-acquired automatic mechanisms – instincts – but on the other hand it gives us a certain degree of control over them. If we feel a bitter taste in our mouth when we eat something bitter, there is nothing we can do about it. Our receptors simply react and the sensation appears. Anger is similar. If something makes us angry, anger pops up and takes hold of us. It is as if it rises up within us and fills us up. Thus, Heidegger says that anger overwhelms us, it takes possession of us.

In seizing the subject, however, they seem to be split in two or doubled. A person can be transported "without themselves", they can be completely "outside themselves", as if they were not even themselves. They do not know how to control themselves; they are not the master of their feelings and thoughts. Rather, they are subjugated to them. We just cannot help it, we just get angry.

Sometimes the anger can be so intense that we really do not even seem to notice what we are doing or saying when we are in the throes of it. Anger, or even amok, takes over our whole mind, our body, and the world we are in. In such an affect, it is as if it is not even us, but someone else, which we often take into account in our evaluation of our act in the affect.

But on the other hand, most of the time a tantrum is not so intense or complex. Most of the time, we can very well distinguish between what our somatic markers are telling us and how we should behave. Our body is telling us that we do not find a given situation, behavior, or phenomenon acceptable. But at the same time, when we are angry, we also perceive that we do not like the situation, the perceived evaluation of the situation. In other words, when we get angry, we are not only the prisoners of a strict reaction to a stimulus, but we also perceive this perception and evaluate it. In this way, anger defies the function performed by a primary emotion or feeling. They are simply reactions to stimuli.

Anger is a special form of reaction. Most somatic markers are designed to provide us with information about the state of the body's receptors. When we get angry, we know we do not like something. We feel resentment as well as a readiness to change state. At the same time, however, anger is one of the emotional states that needs its outward expression to be seen. Anger is meant to be seen. We know that we do not like something, just like we know that we are hungry. We do not need to make an outwardly visible announcement. However, anger is different. It seems that an equally important function of anger, in addition to conveying information to an organism, is its outwardly visible expression. Anger is especially meaningful if we express it. Hidden anger is a contradiction in terms. The primary function of anger is that we make a signal to others (Démuth, 2021).

That hiding anger is not natural is proven by the fact that to keep our anger hidden we need to expend additional energy. We keep ourselves under control, we fight our anger, and we overwhelm our feelings of anger so that our anger is not seen. However, it is natural for anger to be seen.

In this respect, anger is no longer just a feeling, it is also an emotion that needs to be expressed for others to see. When we are angry, our facial appearance changes, our forehead becomes wrinkled, our eyebrows are lowered, we squint... Our muscles stiffen, often we clench our teeth, even our lips – we are simply announcing that we are potentially ready to attack. Since so far, the one we are angry with has overlooked us and ignored us, we raise our voice, use harsh words so that they finally register that we do not like the situation, the action, and the state of affairs. So, anger is mainly directed at another person. It must be clearly expressed and articulated. That we can sometimes suppress or overcome it does not indicate that it has an inwardly directed nature, but only that we can control and regulate it, (as opposed to feeling it) as an outwardly manifested emotional state, as we need.

The Evolutionary Role of Anger

In *How to Do Things with Emotions*, Owen Flanagan (Flanagan, 2021) identifies the evolutionary reasons for the existence of anger in the form of an organism's readiness to defend itself, mobilize, and change its environment. Even relatively simple organisms possess the ability to respond to existential threats by mobilizing their forces and attempting toward off impending danger. Anger is thus one of the mechanisms of self-defense and self-preservation, at least in the sense that it allows us to gather and use energy to prepare for combat or other means of defense. Most animals, however, do not continue this reaction just to mobilize their forces.

As we have already mentioned, an essential part of anger, as an emotion, is that it is expressed toward others. Animals not only express their anger (that they do not like the situation), but also that they are ready to fight. Indeed, part of their defensive strategy is a kind of intimidation, i.e., demonstrating that they are bigger than they look (e.g., puff up their fur), that they are stronger and heavier than they really are. But why do they do this? Simply because they want to intimidate the enemy and deter them from attacking. And it is here that we come to the key evolutionary moment of anger.

The reason we express anger at someone else is not because we could not otherwise defend ourselves. We do not need to express anger in order to attack. On the contrary, by expressing it, we diminish the possible benefits that would result from a surprise attack that would be possible if we felt the anger but did not outwardly express it.

Thus, if we outwardly express anger, thereby forgoing the possibility of a surprise attack and generously affording the adversary an opportunity to prepare for a potential attack, it is not some manifestation of superiority in the form of a handicap (Zahavi, 1975). Quite the contrary, rather, we are trying to avert a possible physical dispute along with the attendant risk of injury or loss in the form of a "diplomatic note".

By outwardly expressing our anger, we announce to those we are angry with that their actions, or the situation they have caused, is no longer acceptable to us. But more than that, we make it clear that to resolve this unacceptable situation, we are prepared to take the risk of that we will lose a relationship, lose favor, or even risk a physical attack and injury, unless a remedy can be found. Thus, an expression of anger is a way to fight back through intimidation.

Susan Riechert, in her research on spider behavior (Riechert, 1986), found that where two approximately equally powerful individuals meet in a conflict of interest, there is an enormous likelihood of a physical altercation. However, the risk of injury and possibly death is associated with a physical attack and combat. Injuring a spider also imposes an additional energy cost, since the injured spider must expend more energy to hunt for food, since it has been injured, and, moreover, it is easier to fall victim to another attack as it is already injured. That said, a real physical encounter is always strenuous and highly risky. It is therefore more sensible to avoid a clash, for example, through intimidation.

Moreover, Riechert found that if the weight difference between the two rivals is large enough, attacks only sporadically occur. The smaller individual will retreat rather than take too great a risk of conflict. This is especially true if the smaller one is an intruder who has tried to acquire the home spider's web. The latter is more often prepared to defend its web as it perceives that it is "in the right", i.e. that it has expended a lot of its energy to weave it. Abandoning it would mean that it would have to expend energy on a new web, with the risk that the situation will be repeated.

If the weight difference is small, the probability of a physical fight increases. Again, however, the home spider has a greater reluctance to leave the battlefield than the intruder. The likelihood and frequency of conflict also increases if there is a scarcity of resources in the environment. In that case, fighting is more efficient, since the energy expenditure to weave a new web is too high, since (due to lack of food) a new web in a new location may not yield enough food and to abandon an existing web may be a waste of precious energy if the new web in a new location fails to provide the same yield. Again, however, the organism that has put in more energy stands to lose more and is more motivated to take the risk of fighting than its opponent. If, however, it assesses the situation as not being worth it, the predatory or marauding strategy may be successful.

The essential feature of the evolution of anger is that it only works if the expression of anger is terrifying enough to cause the recipient to change behavior. If it is not sufficient, the "guilty" person will not be motivated to change their behavior. If, on the other hand, the terror generated by the anger is too great, to the extent that the opponent would rather take the risk of fighting than to endure the terror from the anger, again it will have no effect. The issue, then, seems to be to find the right degree and intensity of anger that can be expressed in equilibrium with the possible consequences that flow from ignoring it.

If Darwin's thesis (Darwin 1859/2002) that it is mainly those organisms that use effective behavioral strategies that survive, it turns out that displays of anger is one of the most effective ways to protect our own interests while eliminating the risks associated with unnecessary physical conflict. Thus, it is an evolutionarily successful strategy. Owen Flanagan argues that, from an evolutionary point of view, as a successful strategy anger will increase in nature (Flanagan, 2018). In particular, those animals that are able to use it effectively survive. Classical philosophical theories of anger (e.g., Aristotle's) link anger to revenge and a desire for retribution. In reality, however, it is a reaction which is intended to reverse a situation or avert danger. The role of anger, therefore, may not only be retaliation; more often it is prevention.

The strategy of expressing anger thus has an inherently social and moral dimension. The social aspect is that it is addressed to others as a signal of fundamental dissatisfaction and the unacceptability of a particular behavior, condition, or situation. Anger presupposes, in principle, that it is directed or addressed to someone.

I primarily address anger toward those to which it belongs. I signal the need to change their undesirable behavior. In doing so, I communicate an important message, the purpose of which is to prevent physical contact.

It can certainly be argued that I can also be angry with myself. This happens when I have not done something I should have. I can be angry when I trip over a stone, I can be angry with the weather, I can be angry with other inanimate objects. Where am I addressing the message in such cases?

The social character of anger toward inanimate objects can be explained in two ways. The first, the easier explanation is with our anger we signal to other people that we are angry about something, and thus we reveal our inner state of mind. This warns them that it is not a good time to address us.

The intersubjective nature of anger, however, is not just about letting others know that I am upset. I would suggest that even in such a form of anger there is a hidden social and particularly moral aspect to my anger. If I am angry with myself, it is because I can perceive a difference between the way I am and the way I ought to be. I address this annoyance at my own failure to myself, that is, toward the one who has failed, from the position of the someone who knows how it should have been. Why do we express it? Sometimes it is to make it obvious to others that we are dissatisfied with our own performance. More often, however, it is that Heideggerian splitting of the subject in its affect. The one who is angry is someone other than the one at whom we are angry. The expression of such anger makes sense to the expressor, less so to the receiver. It is similar when we are angry at inanimate objects.

If I am angry with the weather, a snagged rope, or a rock in the road, I am expressing my conviction and resentment that something is not as it should be. This normative nature of anger, the awareness of how things ought to be, suggests that anger is bound to normativity. What makes us angry is something that has not only defied our will, but it is also something that we have subjectively evaluated as something that is different from how it "ought to be". Thus, the expression of anger is a manifestation of the incongruity of our beliefs about how things ought to be and how they are. This is only meaningful if there is an addressee for the message I wish to send. That addressee may be another person who left the stone in the way, or someone who did not leave the stone in the way, but should know that obstacles should not to be left in the way. It can be someone specific, the world, God, anyone, as we believe that an expression of anger has an effective purpose.

The Ontogenesis of Anger

There are numerous situations when it is not reasonable to express anger. For example, when we assume that our anger will not deter our opponent but will only reveal our weaknesses. If we are angry, we make it clear that we do not have sufficient effective means to change the situation through our own strength without some conflict. If we could do that, why bother to send any signals? If we send them, we feel a certain helplessness. We know that we cannot change the situation through peaceful means alone. We need – we want their assistance. But we probably realize that anger will not help us but rather it will hurt us; so it would be foolish to express it. Therefore, education and experience teach us to handle, manage, and control anger more successfully.

A young child, as soon as it is born, makes its views known through various expressions of anger or its derivatives. Crying, shouting, defiance, or throwing themselves on the ground are all forms through which they express resentment and refuse to cooperate when they do not want to. Over time, however, we gain control over our bodies and learn not to express some of our emotional states or to express them in socially acceptable ways. But it is not just about learning to control ourselves and not express our anger. What we gradually learn is to "read" the situation, to understand that sometimes it is inappropriate to express anger, and we also find there are times when it is good to put it aside or express it in a culturally effective way. Culture and upbringing teach us that anger can also be expressed calmly, that it can be expressed with diplomatic grace, etc. We understand that the presence of anger is unpleasant, not only to us but also to those around us, and the annoyance this causes can handicap us. No one likes it if we are unable to control ourselves, when we are unpleasant, when we make life unpleasant for others. Sometimes an angry person can impress someone because it is obvious that they are not afraid of the consequences of their anger. But most of the time, anger is a manifestation of not being "the master of our own house", of not being a good companion, and of not being able to completely stay in control, because mostly we use anger when we have no other effective remedy.

William Shakespeare (Shakespeare, 1588-1593/2006) describes the anger of Tamora and Timon as an example of this phenomenon. The woman's anger in his plays is childish and hysterical – it is an expression of helpless power. Katherine grimaces and screams, she is snide and vicious, but she cannot come to grips with her situation. We might therefore expect similar anger from Tamora. All the more so because she is a heathen, and therefore a woman uncultured by a Christian upbringing. In contrast, Timon's anger should be calm, steady but deliberate, fully under the control of reason at every moment, without unnecessary affectations, shouting, aware of his powers and competence, but also of the possible consequences. Shakespeare, however, overturns this prejudice. He shows that Tamora can be icily cruel, thoughtful, and deeply aggressive, capable of avenging the monarch. By contrast, it is Timon who succumbs to his supposed power, out of the power itself. He is affectively cruel to the point of punishing an enemy where there is no need to do so, and he reacts inhumanly to Tamora's vengeance when he has her eat her own offspring. Shakespeare brilliantly demonstrates that anger must be controlled, not only in its immediate expression but especially with regard to its consequences. Education and experience often teach us that it is far more effective to curb our anger and use other means to achieve our ends. Where anger is not necessary, because we can achieve the desired result in other ways, it is needless. If we cannot achieve our goals through our own efforts, anger is a cry for help. A cry that announces that we are dependent on someone else to change the situation. Most of the time, we are angry at them because we believe they caused the unacceptable situation and therefore are the only ones who can remedy it.

In her essay *On anger*, Agnes Callard (Callard, 2018) highlights how two common misconceptions associated with anger are incorrect. The first is that anger is a desire for revenge. Callard shows that if someone does something wrong to us, logically nothing is changed if it is put right later. The reason for our anger is that we have been wronged and making things right does not change that. Our anger should therefore, according to her, exist forever, since it is not the disturbance of an objective state, but a disturbance in the relationship between at least two individuals. Therefore, anger should only pass (independently of things) when the original relationship, that has been disturbed, is restored. Certainly, in ordinary life, we feel that perpetual anger is meaningless, especially if the guilty party has repented of their sin, made amends, and credibly promised not to repeat it again. What we are after, according to Callard, is the repair of the relationship. Therefore, it is wrong for us to take justice into our own hands while angry, and make amends. Such corrections can only be about correcting the original wrong, not a correction of the relationship. Taking supposed justice into our own hands is generally not the solution. First, it may be that our anger-accompanied "justice" does not come with all the relevant information and is therefore "unjust". Second, it is sometimes very difficult to determine the right measure of revanche. Logically, we are not looking for an Aristotelian compensatory injustice; therefore, if the injustice were only to result in compensation of losses (I will take from you what you took from me), it would not be any kind of deterrent. Therefore, to redress an injustice, we often reach for retribution with "interest". However, the amount of "interest" can sometimes be very questionable and thus anger can have the exact opposite effect than what we wanted to achieve. Instead of an acknowledgment of guilt and an effort to repair the relationship on the part of the guilty party, there is the perception of a new injustice and a new desire for revenge. Thus, the spiral of vendetta unwinds. The third (and psychologically most important) problem, however, is that in many cases exacting revenge solves nothing at all. Revenge may not soothe the pain, but quite the opposite.

Whereas in the initial perception of anger, there was a feeling of injustice and grief at the fact that someone close to us had dared to harm us, disregard us, or behave in a morally unacceptable way – in exacting revenge we have become like them. We can no longer claim to be the standard for righteousness, no longer the one who is pure and just. We are just the same as the other, whom we reproached with anger for their guilt because we have committed the same act. Moreover, it is clear that we have distorted the essence of our relationship by not allowing them the opportunity to make amends. We did not allow them to return to the relationship. We made amends.

Sure, sometimes the problem is that the other person does not perceive the legitimacy of our anger. Sometimes they do not recognize that we are right. And sometimes they do not care. And this, according to Callard, is at the heart of anger. We perceive that the relationship, as we originally perceived it, has been disrupted and only they can fix it. If they do not, nothing we do will bring them back into the relationship. Trust and gratitude, like apologies, cannot be forced. And if they do, then it is only a formality.

So, what should we do if the other person does not react to our anger and ignores it? There is probably nothing we can do to them. The only thing we can do is to change our attitude or transform our anger.

As Martha Nussbaum (Nussbaum, 2016) shows, perpetual anger is exhausting and inherently harmful. Not only does it leave no room for renewal and improvement of the relationship, but it greatly hurts the person who is angry. Anger consumes energy, it mobilizes us, but at the same time, it is a retreat into the past. It continually throws previous wrongs in our faces and does not allow us to concentrate on something new for the future. If we insist on apologies and cling to satisfaction, we may never get them. Our desire will remain unfulfilled and we will be unhappy. Instead, Nussbaum recommends we transform our anger into something positive. Perhaps into something that will improve our abilities so that in the future we will not find ourselves in a similarly undesirable situation where once again we might become angry. Maybe we should use our anger as a driver to do something to prove to ourselves and the world that we are worthy of love, trust, respect, and relationships. Thus, anger can motivate us to be better, to improve, and to be stronger and more resilient. But again, this has to do with the ability to enter into relationships, not shut ourselves off from them. Only forgiveness can open us to others and it is only through openness, yes even openness to further possible hurt, that we can move on and evolve.

A special kind of anger, therefore, is anger at oneself. Although it may sound illogical, since anger is a reproach to another, a great deal of anger is internally addressed. We are angry that we did not accomplish something, that we were stupid and let ourselves get caught up, betrayed, hurt, and so on. While being angry at someone else can be "solved" by not talking to them anymore, being angry at ourselves is considerably more difficult. Unlike the other guys, we cannot just completely ignore ourselves. Inner remorse, the pain of what hurts is not so easily ignored. They constantly echo; they burn and cannot be banished. So, we look for solutions. Sometimes in what will quell the remorse, sometimes in what will dull our consciousness, sometimes in self-harm to the body that eases the mind. Anger toward oneself can result in self-hatred, serious mental anguish, and even suicide or attempted suicide. One of the greatest arts is the ability to forgive oneself, to recognize one's vulnerability and imperfections, so that we may acknowledge our weaknesses and bring our self-image closer to our true self. Forgiving the other, but especially ourselves, can allow us to move higher, overcome our weaknesses, and make us more resilient in relation to others and ourselves.

The Phylogeny of Anger

If it is the case that we must learn to control, manage, overcome, or even replace anger through forgiveness or by transforming it into something positive, why did it develop in us at all? What evolutionary role does it serve and is it still beneficial?

Owen Flanagan (Flanagan 2018) and many other philosophers, evolutionary psychologists, or biologists will probably highlight its important phylogenetic function, namely, that anger mobilizes an organism, prepares it for a fight, and enables the individual or group to fight back. We have shown in the text that, alongside this, anger has an important moral function in society, and this is threefold. First, by enabling us to perceive a situation or someone as morally and socially unacceptable, i.e., by resisting our willingness to live in a world where unacceptable conditions and rules would prevail. In this sense, anger is an indicator of something wrong in society. It is an indicator of a morally unacceptable contradiction between the way the world is and the way it ought to be.

Second, anger is a morally significant channel of communication. It is an important evolutionarily acquired way to signal our resentment or attitude toward others and is a call for the elimination of evil, unacceptable situations or forms of behavior. Through this, we provide important feedback to help them to understand that their behavior is unacceptable. Therefore, if they wish to continue to work with us, they need to change their attitude or form of behavior. Without such feedback, it would not be possible to improve the world in any meaningful way. It is only when our actions are resisted by something or someone that we are compelled to consider them at all. Sometimes these are purely technical considerations (how to eliminate resistance), but sometimes they are normative and ethical – how to act to make it right. If we do not send any signals, they have no way of knowing that their action is perhaps wrong or cruel. And if they have no way of knowing, how can they improve and how can the world as a whole improve? The road to eternal peace, then, is a road through conflict (Kant).

A third, no less evolutionarily important moral aspect of anger, is its ability to prevent conflict. It is precisely because when angry we signal our attitude, resentment, and readiness to fight for our rights that we prevent a great deal of conflict. Like the *Agelenopsis aperta* spider, we use anger to intimidate our opponents, to announce our resentment and thus the risk of conflict, the importance of something to us in our world, and thus we force the other to consider whether or not it is worth ignoring us. It is strange, but a symbolic (preventive) conflict, in the form of anger, is the best form of prevention of a real physical conflict that would have to follow if we did not symbolically declare our attitude. Paradoxically, anger, which is itself conflict, is the "soft" version of the possible "hard" conflict, and it is only through its persuasiveness that we may be able to prevent real conflict.

Nevertheless, anger acts in a highly ambivalent way in society. Many point out that it is emotionality, and anger in particular, that fosters and causes conflict in society. So, is anger an inhibitor or a catalyst for conflict?

Similarly, as Anjan Chatterjee (Chatterjee 2014) has shown in the case of beauty, which from an evolutionary point of view has played an important role in the selection of fit and suitable genes in the search for mates, evolution does not always go in the same direction as culture. Our evolutionarily acquired intuitive instincts have taught us to seek suitable mates primarily based on physical or other externally perceived indicators of health, fertility, fitness, or other predictors of success in a partnership and ultimately in a greater likelihood of success for our offspring (e. g. Démuthová,

Hudáková, 2023; Démuthová, Minárová, 2023). However, we have succeeded through culture, science, medicine, the availability of food, and many other factors to make those indicators less important, as today even offspring with less-than-optimal genetic predispositions, that for millennia we have learnt to perceive and recognize, are able to survive.

There are similarities with anger. It is clear that it mainly originated as a defensive reaction whose role was to prepare an individual to fight and, on the other hand, to send signals to an opponent to intimidate them and prevent a physical fight. Our ability to "read" anger is thus part of a broader package of our ability to empathize and understand the emotional states of others. It is one of the tools of social survival. An ability to recognize facial movements and identify the specific emotions behind them allows us to anticipate the intentions of a particular individual. And anticipation enables cooperation or, conversely, non-cooperation.

We seem to be evolutionarily pre-equipped to have near-universal expressions and experiences for particular emotions. This allowed our ancestors to understand the facial expression of another member of their own group, their clan, but also the expression of someone from a different tribe, regardless of proximity, distance of kinship, or social relations. The basic expressions of anger, joy, sadness, etc. are, it seems, universal and cross-cultural. However, our coexistence in social communities has also led to the development of another, more effective channel of communication, the development of languages. Languages and their use allow us to communicate even highly subtle semantic distinctions in a very clear way. Moreover, it even allows us to express highly abstract and complicated ideas, and that also with respect to the important temporal localization of intended actions. While anger, expressed in mimicry or gesture, is supposed to be an expression of an immediate threat, through language we can move this threat in time, localizing it for the time when some condition or demand will or will not be fulfilled. We can clarify what we dislike and distinguish the sources of anger from other forms of behavior, situations, or phenomena that do not disturb us so much. This has made language (speech) a more effective, less energy-consuming, and above all more accurately expressive channel of communication, which allows us to eliminate all the unwanted collateral damage that anger expressed emotionally might cause.

Where vocal communication is not effective (when the other person does not understand us or acts as if they do not), we have no choice but to reach for an earlier, more original, form of communication, emotional expressions. We raise our voices, change the cadence of our words, and gesticulate more wildly to send our message when abstract speech has failed. This is how we communicate with our enemies, strangers, and children if we think they might not be able to fully understand what we are saying to them.

Conclusion

Anger is an important evolutionarily evolved state of an organism, which signals: (a) the presumed occurrence of a threatening or undesirable behavior, phenomenon, or situation; (b) the fact that a given situation, phenomenon or behavior, is morally undesirable from our point of view and that it is contrary to our idea of how the world, phenomenon, situation, and behavior, should look like; (c) the readiness to change a given situation, situational behavior through our own behavior (by fighting or refusing contact and cooperation); (d) that it is a fundamentally social, intersubjective, and moral emotional state, which is intended as a message to someone else; (e) that the behavior of others needs to change; and (f) the potential of conflict which hopes to prevent a real physical conflict. Thus, the paradoxical role of anger is to respond to perceived moral evil and thereby make the world a better place by pointing out the unacceptability of evil and a readiness to eliminate it. Often, however, it is our readiness to change the world to our own liking, taking supposed justice into our own hands, our limited rationality, our disregard for each other's perspectives and intentions, and especially the insensitive way in which we express anger, that can cause an increase in conflict and injustice in the world. Therefore, given the social context, the perception of anger, but especially its expression, tends to be socially and culturally influenced, particularly in order to eliminate its undesirable consequences.

Here anger can be likened to a kind of emotional teeth. Their role is to tear, shrink, and eliminate the problem. Eliminating that which is itself inedible in such a form. At the same time, when we bare them we wish to inform the enemy that we are armed with teeth, and that we are ready to use them. However, culture, and especially the use of language, allows us to restrict, control, and even transform our baring of teeth, sometimes even to the point of a kind and acceptable criticism or to express an opinion in an acceptable or perhaps even graceful way. Just as we expose our teeth to view, without fear, when we smile or laugh. We can be diplomatic where there is no need to be frightened. Where they do not understand diplomatic language, there is nothing to do but let them see the possible blood on our fangs.

Given the ever-increasing social aspect of our being in the world, the consequently increased frequency of contact and potential conflict as distances between us shrinks, the number of clashes of interest increases, and the availability of natural resources becomes more limited. It has to be expected that in an ever more densely populated world, there will be more opportunities for the expression of anger. On the other hand, our global society forces us to seek forms of behavior and conflict resolution that do not fatally damage us. The study of anger (political, social, economic, but also personal), the way in which we can control and manage it, but also transform it into something positive, will therefore be an increasingly frequent area of research within the social sciences. Indeed, the evolutionary legacy cannot be completely eliminated, and anger will always somehow emerge. What we can do however, is ensure that there are forms of social regulation and the regulation of its acceptable forms. But these become less necessary in environments where there is less scarcity (we can afford to be more generous in a favorable environment than in an environment with scarce resources), and in environments with less need for collective solutions to individual problems (Démuth 2013). An economically developed, democratic and liberal society will tolerate anger more often and in a better way than a poor or collectivist society (Eriksson et al. 2021). On the other hand, in a society where we most often live and which we prefer, with family, friends, and acquaintances, anger is less frequent and, when it does occur, it is only tolerated if it is bearable. What we seek is the removal of evil but in a kind and gentle manner. So, can evolutionarily hard anger be transformed into a form of kind admonishment?

References

Achs, R. (2020,04,16). Accountability without Vengeance. In *Boston Review*. Retrieved 2024/05/12 from https://www.bostonreview.net/forum_response/rachel-achs-accountability-without-vengeance/

American Psychological Association (2018, April 19). Anger. In *APA Dictionary of Psychology*. Retrieved 2024/05/12 from https://dictionary.apa.org/anger

Bloom, P. (2020,04,16). Choosing Violence. In *Boston Review*. Retrieved 2024/05/12 from https://www.bostonreview.net/forum_response/paul-bloom-choosing-violence/

Bruenig, E. (2020,04,16). The Kingdom of Damage. In *Boston Review*. Retrieved 2024/05/12 from https://www.bostonreview.net/forum_response/elizabeth-bruenig-kingdom-damage/

Butler, J. (inteviewed by Terry, B. M.) (2020). The Radical Equality of Lives. In Callard, A. (2020a) *On Anger*. MIT Press, pp. 85–100.

Cambridge University Press. (n.d.). "Anger" In *Cambridge Dictionary*. Retrieved 2024/05/12 from https://dictionary.cambridge.org/thesaurus/anger

Callard, A. (2017). The Reason to Be Angry Forever. In Myisha Cherry & Owen Flanagan (eds.), *The Moral Psychology of Anger* (pp. 123–138). Rowman & Littlefield International.

Callard, A. (2020a) *On Anger*. MIT Press.

Callard, A. (2020,04,16b). The Philosophy of Anger. In *Boston Review*. Retrieved 2024/05/12 from http://bostonreview.net/forum/agnes-callard-philosophy-anger

Callard, A. (2020,04,16c). The Wound Is Real. In *Boston Review*. Retrieved 2024/05/12 from https://www.bostonreview.net/forum_response/agnes-callard-wound-real/

Cameron, D., & Spring, V. (2020,04,16). The Social Life of Anger. In *Boston Review*. Retrieved 2024/05/12 from https://www.bostonreview.net/forum_response/daryl-cameron-victoria-spring-social-life-anger/

Chatterjee, A. (2014). *The Aesthetic Brain How We Evolved to Desire Beauty and Enjoy Art*. Oxford University Press.

Damasio, A. (1999). *The Feeling of What Happens: Body, Emotion and the Making of Consciousness*. Vintage.

Darwin, Ch. (1859/2002). *On the Origin of Species by Means of Natural Selection, or the Preservation of Favoured Races in the Struggle for Life*. In Van Wyhe, John, ed. Darwin Online: On the Origin of Species, 2002. Retrieved 2024/05/01 from: https://darwin-online.org.uk/EditorialIntroductions/Freeman_OntheOriginofSpecies.html.

Démuth, A. (2024a). *Anger as A/Moral Emotion.* Peter Lang.

Démuth, A. (2024b). O hneve, alebo čo ponúka Heideggerova filozofia afektivity. [On Anger, or What Heidegger's Philosophy of Affectivity Offers]. *Filosofický časopis.* 72(3), 415-429.

Démuth, A. (2013). *Game Theory and Problem of Decision Making.* Towarzystwo Słowaków w Polsce.

Démuth, A. (2021). Hnev ako sociálna a morálna emócia. [Anger as a Sotial and Moral Emotion]. In *Bratislavské právnické fórum 2021: Kríza autorít a hodnôt súčasnej spoločnosti.* Bratislava: Právnická fakulta UK, pp. 23-30.

Démuthová, S. Hudáková, A. (2023). Attractive human face as a communication tool: Age and gender specifics of the attractiveness of sexually dimorphic features in facial composites. *Communication Today.* 14(2), 90-102; https://doi.org/10.34135/communicationtoday.2023.Vol.14.No.2.7.

Démuthová, S., Minárová, D. (2023). The Evolutionary Principles of the Attractiveness of Symmetry and Their Possible Sustainability in the Context of Research Ambiguities. *Brain : broad research in artificial intelligence and neuroscience.* 14(1), 515-534; https://doi.org/10.18662/brain/14.1/433.

Descartes, R. (1649/2002). *The Passions of the Soul* (Translated by Stephen Voss). Hackett.

Dixon, T. (2020). What Is the History of Anger a History of? *Emotions: History, Culture, Society.* 4(1), 1-34. Retrieved 2023/11/30 from https://brill.com/view/journals/ehcs/4/1/article-p1_2.xml?ebody=full html-copy1

Ekman, P. (1999). Basic Emotions. *Handbook of Cognition and Emotion, 98,* (45-60).

Eriksson, K., Strimling, P., & Gelfand, M. *et al.* (2021). Perceptions of the Appropriate Response to Norm Violation in 57 Societies. *Nature Communications 12,* 1481; https://doi.org/10.1038/s41467-021-21602-9.

Flanagan, O. (2018). Introduction: The Moral Psychology of Anger. In Myisha Cherry & Owen Flanagan (eds.), *The Moral Psychology of Anger* (pp. vii–xxxi). Rowman & Littlefield.

Flanagan, O. (2021). *How to Do Things with Emotions.* Princeton University Press.

Gärdenfors, P. (2000). *Conceptual Spaces: The Geometry of Thought.* The MIT Press.

Greenstein, M., & Franklin, N. (2020). Anger Increases Susceptibility to Misinformation. *Experimental Psychology, 67*(3), 202-209. https://doi.org/10.1027/1618-3169/a000489

Gilam, G., & Hendler, T. (2017). Deconstructing Anger in the Human Brain. *Current Topics in Behavioral Neurosciences, 30,* 257-273. https://doi.org/10.1007/7854_2015_408

"Hate" 4/19/2018). In *APA Dictionary of Psychology.* Retrieved 2024/05/12 from https://dictionary.apa.org/hate

"Hatred" (n. d.). In Reber, A.S. (1995) *In Penguin Dictionary of Psychology.* London: Penguin Books.

"Hatred" (2024). In *Merriam-Webster Dictionary*. Retrieved 2024/05/12 from https://www.merriam-webster.com/dictionary/hatred

Heidegger, M. (1996). *Nietzsche I*. GA. Bd. 6.1. Vittorio Klostermann.

Herman, B. (2020,04,16). What's Past Is Prologue. In *Boston Review*. Retrieved 2024/05/12 from https://www.bostonreview.net/forum_response/barbara-herman-whats-past-prologue/

Cherry, M. (2020,04,16). More Important Things. In *Boston Review*. Retrieved 2024/05/12 from https://www.bostonreview.net/forum_response/myisha-cherry-more-important-things/

Jagmohan, D. (2020,04,16). Anger and the Politics of the Oppressed. In *Boston Review*. Retrieved 2024/05/12 from https://www.bostonreview.net/forum_response/desmond-jagmohan-anger-and-politics-oppressed

Konstans, D. (2020). A History of Anger. In Callard, A. (2020a) *On Anger*. MIT Press, pp. 101–111.

Miller, M. M., Williams, A. E., Scott, E. L., Trost, Z., & Hirsh, A. T. (2022). Anger as a Mechanism of Injustice Appraisals in Pediatric Chronic Pain. *The Journal of Pain*, 23(2), 212–222. https://doi.org/10.1016/j.jpain.2021.07.005

Merriam-Webster. (n.d.). Hate. In *Merriam-Webster.com Dictionary*. Retrieved 2024/04/15 from https://www.merriam-webster.com/dictionary/hate

Muellner, L. (1996). *The Anger of Achelles*. Retrieved 2023/04/15 from http://nrs.harvard.edu/urn-3:hul.ebook:CHS_MuellnerL.The_Anger_of_Achilles.1996.

Na'aman, O. (2020,04,16). Against Moral Purity. In *Boston Review*. Retrieved 2024/05/12 from https://www.bostonreview.net/forum_response/oded-naaman-against-moral-purity/

Nussbaum, M. C. (2016). *Anger and Forgiveness: Resentment, Generosity, Justice*. Oxford University Press.

Nussbaum, M. C. (2020). Victim Anger and Its Cost. In Callard, A. (2020a) *On Anger*. MIT Press, pp. 112–131.

Oberding, A. (2020). Rightous Incivility. In Callard, A. (2020a) *On Anger*. MIT Press, pp. 112–131.

Oster, U. (2014). Emotions between Physicality and Acceptability. A Contrast of the German Anger Words Wut and Zorn. *Onomázein*, (30), 286–306. https://doi.org/10.7764/onomazein.30.19.

Philips, W. (2020). Whose Anger Counts? In Callard, A. (2020a) *On Anger*. MIT Press, pp. 132–147.

Pisárčiková, M. (Ed.) (2004). *Synonymický slovník slovenčiny* [Synonymous Dictionary of Slovak]. Veda.

Potegal, M., & Novaco, R.W. (2010). A Brief History of Anger. In: Michael Potegal, Gerhard Stemmler, & Charles Spielberger (eds.) *International Handbook of Anger*. Springer, https://doi.org/10.1007/978-0-387-89676-2_2

Plutchik, R. (1982). A Psychoevolutionary Theory of Emotions. *Social Science Information*. 21(4–5), pp. 529–553. doi:10.1177/053901882021004003.

Prinz, J. (2020,04,16). How Anger Goes Wrong. In *Boston Review*. Retrieved 2024/05/12 from https://www.bostonreview.net/forum_response/jesse-prinz-how-anger-goes-wrong/

Pubmed (2024). "Anger". Retrieved 2024/05/12 from https://pubmed.ncbi.nlm.nih.gov/?term=anger

Reber, A. S. (1995). "Anger". In *Dictionary of Psychology*. Penguin.

Riechert, S. E. (1986). Spider fights: A Test of Evolutionary Game Theory. *American Scientist*, 47, 604–610.

Shakespeare, W. (1588–1593/2006). *Titus Andronicus*. (Translated by Martin Hilský), Evropský literární klub.

Staicu, M. L., & Cuțov, M. (2010). Anger and Health Risk Behaviors. *Journal of Medicine and Life*, 3(4), 372–375.

"Thumos" (n. d.), In: Thayer, J. H. (n. d.). *Thayer's Greek-English Lexicon of the New Testament*. Retrieved 2024/04/15 from: https://biblehub.com/greek/2372.htm

Twiss, Ch. (15.10.2023). Understanding Why Anger Is a Secondary Emotion? Retrieved 2024/04/15 from https://www.choosingtherapy.com/anger-is-a-secondary-emotion/

Van Doren, N., & Soto, J. A. (2021). Paying the Price for Anger: Do Women Bear Greater Costs?. *International Journal of Psychology : Journal International de psychologie, 56*(3), 331–337. https://doi.org/10.1002/ijop.12724

Walsh, T., R. (2005). *Fighting Words and Feuding Words: Anger and the Homeric Poems (Greek Studies: Interdisciplinary Approaches)* Lexington Books. Retrieved 2023/11/30 from https://chs.harvard.edu/read/walsh-thomas-r-fighting-words-and-feuding-words-anger-and-the-homeric-poems/

Wang, F., & Pereira, A. (2016). Neuromodulation, Emotional Feelings and Affective Disorders. *Mens Sana Monographs, 14*(1), 5–29. https://doi.org/10.4103/0973-1229.154533.

Weiblen, R., Mairon, N., Krach, S., Buades-Rotger, M., Nahum, M., Kanske, P., Perry, A., & Krämer, U. M. (2021). The Influence of Anger on Empathy and Theory of Mind. *PloS one, 16*(7), e0255068. https://doi.org/10.1371/journal.pone.0255068

Williams, R. (2017). Anger as a Basic Emotion and Its Role in Personality Building and Pathological Growth: The Neuroscientific, Developmental and Clinical Perspectives. *Frontiers in Psychology* 8:1950. doi: 10.3389/fpsyg.2017.01950

Yarns, B. C., Cassidy, J. T., & Jimenez, A. M. (2022). At the Intersection of Anger, Chronic Pain, and the Brain: A Mini-Review. *Neuroscience and biobehavioral reviews*, 135, 104558. https://doi.org/10.1016/j.neubiorev.2022.104558

Zahavi, A. (1975). Mate Selection—A Selection for a Handicap. *Journal of Theoretical Biology. 53* (1). Elsevier BV: 205–214.

Guilt
Persons in Web of Guilt. Guilt in Net of Interpretations

Ľubomír Batka

> *In ancient times, people were troubled by transience, in the Middle Ages by guilt, and in modern times by meaninglessness.*
>
> P. Tillich
> The Courage to Be, 1952

The meaning of good and evil depends on metaphysical assumptions about the existence of moral good or evil. In his debates with Manicheans and Pelagians, the Church Father Augustine defended the idea that evil has no being. Evil deeds turn away from "highest good" (sumum bonum) toward nothingness (Ricoeur, 1974, vol. ii., 140-161). Evil is privation of good (privatio boni). It is possible to say: "I do things that are evil", but speaking about deeds as evil misleads to a conclusion that a person performing such act is an "evildoer" and thus an "evil person", This obscures the notion of guilt (Batka, 2023).

Guilt is related to norms preserving or promoting interpersonal relationships. If they promote a relationship to a person, they are described as "right", in case they cause violation, they are "wrong". A negative action is "wrongdoing" toward a person since it crosses the intentions of a relationship drawn by a norm. A person not respecting the "border line" is a "transgressor". The guilt originates from a wrongdoing toward a person by transgressing a norm. In this article, we describe actions causing guilt as "wrongdoing" and "transgression", not necessarily "evil deeds".

We begin with a thought experiment: what would human life look like without guilt? There is no guilt where there is no consciousness about the impact of deeds. A life without understanding of the effect might resemble to a paradise, or as a state of "Dreaming Innocence" (P. Tillich). It would be a life of spiritual emptiness, some sort of preconscious adhering to a pack of other singularities. Before "historical man", one can only speak of "animals" that did not yet have history. With Jürgen Moltmann we can say, "A cow is always a cow. It does not ask, 'What is a cow? Who am I.' Only man asks such questions, and indeed clearly has to ask them about himself and his being. This is his question. His question follows him in hundreds forms" (Moltmann, 1974, 1). If everything is equally valid, everything becomes indifferent.

If there is nonexistence of guilt, it would be impossible to judge the quality of interpersonal relations. Nonexistence of guilt implies an absolute freedom toward other people, without any fear of rejection, since without guilt, no punishment on an objective or subjective level exists. Punishment would be just another act of violence without the framework of justice. In such freedom, no regulation of emotions like anger, hate, and disgust is necessary since there is no fear of violating or losing a relationship to another person. Such emotions would be natural, but not "damaging". All intentions of will can be pursued. Every person would be exposed to unpredictable violence. Guilt would not hinder the loss of respect for other people, for their feelings and dignity: domination and subjugation would become the normal case. There would be radical liberty in choosing individual goals and means, but without duty, responsibility, accountability, and liability to another person. Where there is no victim, there is no guilt and thus no fear about losing lasting relationships.

Unrestricted freedom in choosing goals and means allows only short-time and short-lived projects, which means less innovation, planning, and slow progress. It would be a lonely life, a sort of nomadic life, with few interactions and undeveloped social structures. Life without guilt is a free, intensive, and passionate life, perhaps a life of alfa males, or the Jungian "explorers" or "heroes". It would be a short life and perhaps short for the entire human race.

This negative picture can be met with the opposite question: Is guilt useful for the survival and functioning of an individual or human society?

In What Sense Is Guilt Useful for Human Society?

It might be tempting to quickly assert a utility in guilt. However, there is a danger of utilitarian calculation of guilt: the more guilt there is, the larger good for the largest possible amount of people. As a matter of fact, in Utilitarianism, guilt does not play a role: "Trait guilt will have no association with utilitarian judgment" (Choe, Min, 2011, 584). The principle of utility looks forward to the future, not to actions done in the past.

Guilt is not helpful in a direct way. Individual feelings of guilt do not make the situation of others better. Life of others is made better by positive conduct, promoting interpersonal relations (De Hooge, 2019). Guilt is a capacity to recognize the effect of one's actions on other people and to feel them as negative. It is an ability "to acknowledge" and "to feel" the wrongdoing and pain experienced by the other person. In his analysis of Totalitarianism, T. Zálešák concluded: "Where both the killer and the victim, as well as the relationship between them, are radically depersonalized, there can be no question of guilt and responsibility. ... Where there is no moral person and individuality, there is neither guilt nor the feeling of wrong, resulting from the consciousness of personal harm" (Zálešák, 2005, 106). Guilt is a sort of empathy a posteriori: as respect to the experience of the other and an acknowledgment of negative effects. Against the "I will for me!" of Friedrich Nietzsche, one wants to grant space for the other person as an equal person in dignity and rights.

Guilt is a negative response to an action that was not supposed to be done since it contradicts the interest and violates the dignity of others. Expectations of what ought or ought not to be done have their value in the connection to an interpersonal relationship. Guilt preserves moral conduct on an individual level and intrapersonal level and forms relations and societal structures protected in a legal framework.

Guilt can have a role in motivating self-control before the action, avoiding negative consequences, or preserving valuable relationships. Long-lasting relationships and cooperation are possible through concepts of justice, right, and wrong. According to Meteňkanyč: "Justice and emotions are an important part of organisational life, characterizing and informing organizational procedures as well as acting as ommunication systems that help individuals navigate through the basic problems that arise in social relations" (Meteňkanyč, 2023, 144). Law and morality call to responsibility and duty, which leads to societal progress in the long run. On the other side, the development of human rights increases the possibilities of wrongdoing.

Persons in Web of Guilt

According to Dorothea Sitzler-Osing, guilt can be seen from four possible points of view: the point of view of the person as victim, or as transgressor, the deed (transgression), and the normative system (Sitzler-Osing, 1999, 572–577). Each perspective correlates to another part and they are often intertwined. Right and wrong measures deeds and goals as wrong on the side of a transgressor, or one can describe his own experience and situation as harmful (victim). A norm makes it possible to judge and proclaim guilt between two persons. The question of validity of the normative system used for making judgments about guilt is relevant too.

(1) Eliminatory perception of guilt accentuates the "deed-victim" relation. The subjective guilt of an individual is not in the foreground. Guilt exists objectively in an unfortunate situation. The question about guilt becomes vivid in the occurrence of bad fortune. Suffering, bad luck, sickness, and death result from the existing sphere of guilt. Questions about transgression caused by tribe, family, forefathers, and neighbors arise. Rituals seek to eliminate primarily the existing sphere of guilt (religiously interpreted as flaw, Makel, poškvrna) causing such bad fortune.

(2) Causative perception of guilt accentuates the relation between "normative system-victim". Who is responsible and guilty? What is the reason for condemnation? (αἰτία, causa in legal language). It can appear as well in situations where the normative system is not explicit. The causa can be religiously interpreted as evil spirits, demons, or, like in questions of theodicy, God.

(3) Compensatory perception of guilt concentrates on the perspective "normative system-trespasser". A person is a wrongdoer and becomes a debtor (Schuldner, dlžník, vinník). The guilt (ὀφείλω, debitum, reatus) arises by diversion from a normative system, by not doing what was expected, not fulfilling duty, and by transgressing the norm. Typical compensatory perception of guilt can be found in the Roman legal system. In religion, the term "sin" is used widely ("forgive us our sins/debts"). Questions of injustice and compensation become dominant. Guilt and punishment are nearly identical (i.e., concupiscence in the teaching of Augustine, or the interpretation of original sin as original

debt/guilt). Rituals of penance and confession, ascetism are used to redeem the guilt.

(4) Confessory perception of guilt looks at the "deed-trespasser" connection. Wrong actions make a person transgressor and create guilt. The will and decision (dolus) of a transgressor play an important role in the recognition of guilt. Important means of dealing with this kind of guilt are conscience, self-recognition, confession of guilt, and change of will (metanoia). Confession of guilt can form individual piety. It can be often found in Greek philosophical thinking by Homer, Aristotle, Philo Josephus, as ἁμαρτία (dolus, culpa, peccatum) against divinity, other people, own body. In the background is the idea of missing the right action or to make something wrong according to gods, ethos, and law.

In all four instances, guilt arises in a relationship of two (or more) subjects. The Greek philosophical confessory and the ancient causative conceptions were partly pushed back by the compensatory character of guilt in the Christian teaching on (original) sin. In the sacrament of penance, the confession of sin remained dominant. In Christian religion, the objective guilt toward God developed into a universalistic doctrine on original sin and subjective guilt was radicalized in the practice of (sacrament) of penance. Guilt was expanded not only to moral actions but even to thoughts, words, intentions, and wishes ("movements of the hearth") before an action occurred.

The fourfold characters of guilt elaborated by Karl Jaspers is well known and does not need to be elaborated in this chapter at length. In 1947 Jaspers published his lectures with a title: *"Die Schuldfrage: Von der politischen Haftung Deutschlands"*, the same year translated into English as *"The Question of German Guilt"*. He distinguished political, criminal, moral, and metaphysical guilt. Criminal guilt results from crimes committed by individuals and can be proved by objective facts. Political guilt is borne by every citizen of the state because everybody is responsible for the way he is governed. Moral guilt derives from the human ability to make moral judgments. It is strictly personal; nobody from outside can make a judgment about moral transgression (except a very close person who really cares). Each person must face his or her moral responsibility for all their deeds. A collective can be guilty, but guilt can only be felt by a person. Metaphysical guilt comes from the solidarity among humans in acknowledging the impossibility of overcoming or completely eradicating injustice in the world. Metaphysical guilt reveals a lack of absolute solidarity with other people. Only God can judge this kind of guilt (Jaspers, 2000, 25–27).

Paul Ricoeur in his famous treatise "*Symbolik des Bösen. Phänomenologie der Schuld*" approached the question of guilt from the point of analysis of symbols related to "evil" (containing three levels of development). Symbols express the fundamental human experience and return people to the state of beginning. The way of creative interpretation of symbols leads to deeper awareness of the meaning and better understanding. Guilt can be approached from three cultural contexts: (1) Rational thinking: in ethical-legal reflection about culpability and responsibility by the Greeks. (2) Zeal for inwardness: in ethical-religious reflection about the sensitive and unsensitive consciousness by the Jews. (3) Existential: in psycho-theological reflection about the pains of consciousness under the condemnation of the law by Apostle Paul (Ricoeur, 1971, vol. ii., 117–118). These three contexts are hard to reconcile in one unity. In the phenomenological analysis of Ricoeur, the notion of "human fallibility" incorporates the movement of "breach" (breaking away) and of "resumption" (being accepted back). It's about this "double movement through which guilt releases itself from flaws and sin and captures their primal symbolism" (ebenda, 118). Guilt refers to the subjective element of the wrongdoing. Sin is its ontological moment.

Ricoeur's profound analysis deserves a closer look. In the rationalistic, ethical-legal attribution of guilt, the personal relationship between God and man, respectively, the covenant, do not play a role. Important is the relationship to the state, its legislation, and the structure of criminal law (In ancient Greek all of them can have minimal sacral value.). A question of guilt was fundamental for the public justice. The criminal law in Greece and Rome developed methods to distinguish guilt in various grades. A person can be more guilty or less guilty, and thus a just punishment must reflect this subjective grade of guiltiness. The "just" and "unjust", as well as the "injustice suffered", can be sanctioned by limited and measured satisfaction. The process of limiting and measuring the punishment is the process of measuring the guilt: "Thus the distinction in degrees of guilt, which among the Jews is discovered more in personal reflection within the communal confession, is among the Greeks correlative to a development of criminal law" (ebenda, 130). In the development of Greek Law, punishment was less and less a repression by society. The justice (dike) of the state delivered punishment as satisfaction for the injured party and as a pedagogical-corrective instrument. For this process, the psychological aspect of guilt was not important. The distinction between "deliberate" and "unwillingly" developed fully by Aristotle in his "*Nicomachean Ethics*" considers internal psychology of the transgressor. This distinction is an instrument used by courts. Special attention was given to the unwilling killing that happened by sport-games or in war, since the civic context of those deeds was important.

The second context analyzed by Ricoeur was the "zeal for inwardness", in which the question of guilt depends on the sensitive – "scrupulous" – conscience. Jewish monotheism has a strict ethical character. Simultaneously, Tora is understood exclusively historically as part of one elected nation. Best examples for this attitude were the "Pharisees" in ancient Judaism: "The Pharisee's closed and consistent heteronomy is rooted in the 'historical' character of monotheism, which the legislators ... placed under the authority of Moses" (ebenda, 136). The Pharisees are "men of the Torah", the educators of the Jewish people, the purest representatives of a fundamental type of moral experience in which every person can recognize itself of the possibilities of its own humanity. They want to apply the Torah in most detailed way to all areas of life: ritual, ethics, family, community, criminal law, and economics. "Scruple" is a general rule of behavior that is adopted consistently and with personal consent. The scrupulous conscience is heteronomous; it finds happiness in doing everything what is seen as God's instructions. Rituals confirm conscience in its will to obey the law, which ultimately leads to ritualization of ethics. If this fails, the conscience suffers strong personal guilt and intensive polarity between the "just" and the "wicked" (ebenda, 148). Sin is a transgression, "subjectively, guilt is understood as a loss of a degree of value. It is the ultimate ruin" (ebenda, 150). Zeal for inwardness sharpens the understanding of guilt, leading either to "fanatism" or "encapsulation". In both instances there is a dividing line between those who observe the law and those who do not, between the "pure" and "not-pure", between the "separated" (Pharisees) and the "rest". The opposite to the scrupulous conscience is "hypocrisy".

The third context in Ricoeur's analysis represents the psycho-theological reflection about the pains of guilty – consciousness, of Apostle Paul (or later Augustine, Luther).[8]

It stems from the experience of man's powerlessness to meet the total demands of the Jewish Law. The commandments are "innumerable", and perfection is "infinite". This is the "hell of guilt". The truly new in Pauline theology is that the Jewish Law itself is the source of sin. Instead of leading to righteousness, it creates sin and guilt. Beyond the "juridical" and "scrupulous" understanding of guilt, in this psycho-theological reflection, the very will to be righteous through law becomes "sin". The new quality of evil is the "will to save oneself by fulfilling the law". Striving for one's own righteousness combines "sin", "desire", and "zeal for the law" (ebenda, 163). The opposite of guilt is the freedom (that comes in the free gift of justification through faith alone). Existence without "freedom" is subjected to "slavery", the dominion of the "flesh", and is doomed to "death". In juridical understanding, "death" is the punishment for guilt. In psycho-theological understanding "death" is produced by "sin" according to an "organic law of Dasein" (ebenda, 163). This was not an original "ontological structure", but it became a subsequent "order of existence". Such deepening development of the feeling of guilt in the emergence of self-righteousness and the curse attached to it reinterprets the experience of scruple: "What had not been felt as guilt ... now becomes guilt. Even the endeavor to reduce sin through observance becomes sin" (ebenda, 165). The feeling of guilt crumbles under the "radical demand" and sees the never-ending "multiplicity of regulations". The endless self-accusation does not happen in a court with a counterpart (judge/God). The "curse of law" transforms the feeling of guilt into a juridical language. However, the tribunal, condemnation, and sanction happen in singularity of the self. The result is the self-loathing, self-humiliation, restless self-observation, growing isolation, and lastly the "sin of despair". "This is the sin of all

---

8 For differences between Paul and Luther cf. Althaus, 1963, 54–67. For a comparison of Augustine and Luther, cf. Jenson, 2006, 79–83.

sins: no longer transgression, but despairing and desperate will to lock oneself in the circle of prohibition and desire. In this sense it is desire for death" (ebenda, 169, see S. Kierkegaard).

Later we return to Ricoeur's analysis of the symbols of "sin". His work shows that historically, Christian teaching on sin is a synthesis of Jewish thinking and Greek culture. An excellent example gives the Greek translation of the Bible (Septuagint, LXX). In the translation of a differentiated Hebrew terminology of sin (and guilt) into Greek, some aspects of sin and guilt got lost, another were developed further. A short look at the greatest variety of terminology related to sin (and guilt) in the collection of Hebrew and Greek texts of the Bible will enlighten deeper understanding of sin and guilt.

Sin, Guilt, and Punishment in Biblical Terminology

The Biblical sense of guilt is indivisibly connected with the understanding of sin (Knierim, 2001). This is particularly obvious in the holistic thinking of the ancient Orient. In Hebrew texts, the deed and its consequence are not separated: the beginning, the middle, and the end are dynamic unity.

The best example is the Hebrew term "Avon" (עָוֹן). It unites transgression, conscious, intentional offence, the guilt, and the punishment for guilt in one (Koch, 1992, 49-50). Translating Biblical passages presents a challenge for translators: a plea for forgiveness of sins, means likewise a plea for forgiveness of guilt and the forgiveness of the punishment (cf. Ps 32,5).

The strongest and most central Hebrew term for sin is "pescha" (פֶּשַׁע). It means crime in legal meaning, but likewise a breach of the covenant with God (cf. Jes 1, 2-3). This is not surprising, since in ancient Israel the covenant with Gods included legal social norms. Transgression is a breach of the covenant with God. Theft and homicide sanctioned by criminal law are equally interpreted as breach of contractual relationships. The connection of sin (against God) and crime (against a person) is very strong in this term. In the Bible, special severity is given to crimes in the context of the family (cf. Dtn 22). The guilt rest in the unlawful break away from the covenant, in breaking away from the community, or in breaking of the property of another person (Koch, 1992, 31–41, cf. German "Verbrechen").

According to Ricoeur, the symbol of "rebellion" behind these words expresses the less formal and most existential symbol for sin. The importance of covenant as fundamental for the understanding of sin confirms Ricoeur as well: "Sin is a religious entity before it is ethical: it is not the violation of an abstract rule – a value – but the violation of a personal bond. So we cannot fathom the meaning of sin on its own, but only together with the meaning of this primordial bond that is Spirit and Word" (Ricoeur, 1971, vol. ii., 63, 79).

The third most important Old Testament term is "chata" (אָטָה), literally means "to go off the right path", not to fulfill a promise, or "missing the mark" (f.E. by shooting bow and arrow). It describes a wrong relationship with God or a wrong relationship in a community (cf. 2Sam 12, 13). Translation would be "to fail", "failure", and "fault". It integrates the aspect of "not getting it right". The primary "goal" is not the norm of a normative system. Again, it is a relationship in a community among people (adultery, sexual offense, social exploitation of widows, orphans, strangers) or between a person and God. And again, this term is holistic. The consequence of the failure is included: the term designates the punishment for the transgression as well (Koch, 1992, 44–48). For the Greeks, the symbol of the "path" – the "crooked", "winding path" – was less common than for the Hebrews: "The symbol of error or wandering, which is more tailored to the problem of truth than to that of ethical obedience, takes its place" (Ricoeur, 1971, vol. ii., 139).

"Sin" has 26 expressions in the Old Testament (f.E. evil/ra, mistake/šgagah, violence/hamas, lie/šeker), and the most common ones refer to various aspects of human action and a way of life in a covenantal relationship to God or in a community of other people. The most radical term, the "total rebellion against God" (injustice, rascha, רָשָׁע) stands against "justice" (הָקְדָצ) that exists only in a covenant with God. The Hebrew thinking is not as legalistic as it might appear from afar. The covenant is a way of life, not a set of norms. Religious morality and law in the Old Testament have a personal character (Kašný, 2017, 15). Prohibitions and commands in the Bible are formulated in the second person singular or plural and bind the individual. The discussion about the number of "commandments" to perform an act and about "prohibitions" to abstain from an act played an important role later, in Rabbinic literature.

In his study to the use of the terminology related to sin, R. Koch concluded that the great variety of the Biblical Hebrew was in the Greek translation of Bible (Septuagint, LXX) reduced to only six Greek terms (Koch, 1992, 31-43, Bauer, 1971, Panczová, 2012). Among the hamartiological terminology of the New Testament, the strongest term is the "asebeia" (ασέβεια), designating the error in the cult, negation of religious life, acting against the religion, but also impiety or blasphemy, godless thinking and acting. For Apostle Paul, it described the pagan religion. "Hybris" (ὕβρις) describes pride, abuse, and injury to the honor of Gods. The term "parabasis" (παράβασις) means the transgression of the law and is stronger than "paraptoma" (παραπτώμα) to make a mistake, to step aside, often on plural, as well as collective (in German Vergehen, Verfehlung, Felhtritt). "Ofeilo" (ὀφείλω) connects economical and moral obligations. In the Our Father prayer (Forgive us or "debts"), the aramaic "hôb" connects those two aspects as well (Crüsemann 1992, 92). The most widely used term is "hamartia" (ἁμαρτία). It is related to "hamartano" (ἁμαρτάνω), close to Hebrew "chata" meaning "to miss the mark". Similarly to Hebrew thinking, "hamartia" combines the deed as well as the result of the deed (guilt). It expresses the circle of sin and punishment, blindness, which leads to missing the goal and to further sin (cf. R 1, 28-32, 1K 6, 9-10, G 5, 19-21). It is both a state and a situation, as well as the opposite of the truth (J 9, 41). It is a tragic failure. The symbol of "wandering astray" and "to get lost" (f.E. in the Parable of the lost sheep LK 15, 1-7) speaks about the whole situation of a person, not about the moment of getting lost. This means, it is close to the modern term "alienation" or "to be thrown in" (Ricoeur, 1971, vol. ii., 87).

Further important development in thinking about sin and guilt is related to the practice of penance. By the 3rd century, a system of public penance has developed. Originally, the penance could be undergone only once in a lifetime, which led to postponement of penance until the death. A new system was developed in the 7th century. Penance remained public; however, the confession of sins was secret. The private penance was confirmed by the mandate *"Omnis utriusque sexus"* (1215), which commanded every Christian of the age of discretion to confess all his sins at least once a year to the priest (Cross, 1997, 1250). Penitential Book, Confessor´s Handbook and mendicant orders, as well as other monks fostered the spread of private penance. Penance (poena) was a sort of punishment for the sinner and satisfaction here on earth. First in the 20th century, after Vatican II, did reconciliation and amendment of life become central aspects of the sacrament.

Guilt arose by transgression of a commandment of God or the Church. Penance was a precondition for further participation in religious practice in the Church and sacraments. Guilt could be alleviated by an internal or external act of confession associated with the process of self-knowledge and an expression of will. The Sacrament of Penance in the Medieval Church of the West consisted of three parts: contritio, confessio, satisfactio. A widely debate raised the question of the intensive remorse of the heart, feeling of guilt (contrition vs. attrition). Only sin that was confessed could be absolved. Penitential books helped to recognize the various transgression of deed, and of omission of good. Satisfaction was an instrument to confirm the sincerity of the repentance. Church punishments should motivate from abstaining from further transgressions (peccata acutalia) and were a measure of Church discipline (Pelikan, 1985, 128, 131. Ohst, 1995, 240).

According to Thomas Aquinas, the knowledge of man's sin is derived from the observation of moral failures in man's life. Actions are sinful because they are bad in themselves. The unnaturalness of the deed is rationally understandable. Original sin is the corruption (vitium) into which every person is born. The guilt (reatus) of a person only arises from a sinful act, for which a person freely decided and bears responsibility for it. A sinful act is morally bad and a person could (should) have avoided it. Thanks to the natural faculties strengthened by the grace of God, the sinner's will is able to will what reason knows to be good. Through an internal or external act of confession, the sinner is reintegrated into religious life. Regret for sin, confession of guilt, and the effort to change one's life are manifested in repentance (poenitentia) (Pesch, 1988, 257–260, Cf. Aquinas STh I-II, q. 71, a.6).

The development of the Reformation in 16th century is firmly connected with the criticism of the medieval practice of repentance (poenitientiam agere). Against the general perception, it was not the trade with indulgences itself that moved Luther. His concern was about emptying penance to a mere sacramental act (ritual) that infuses grace and proclaims forgiveness of sins just by mere action (in opere operato), without a sincere feeling of guilt.

Luther, an observant Augustine Eremite mendicant friar developed a new theology of repentance (Schwarz, 1968). In his famous *"Ninety-Five Theses"*, Luther started in the first thesis: "When our Lord and Master Jesus Christ said 'Repent', he willed the entire life of believers to be one of repentance" (LW 31, 25–26). By "repent" (poenitentiam agree), Luther meant the Greek "metanoeite", which means "to regret". A better Latin translation would be "transmentamini", meaning "to pass from one state of mind to another, to arrive at a change of mind". Luther criticized the medieval debates about the size and sufficiency of regret, as well as the question of distinguishing between two types of contrition (contritio and attritio). Luther expected a deep recognition of guilt and a deep sorrow. He experienced the impossibility of confessing all sins. The time of confession should not be prescribed by Church but left open to the desire of conscience troubled by guilt. Further, Luther rejected satisfaction due to the widely spread misconception that a person deserves the forgiveness of sins from God exactly due to satisfactory deeds. Lastly, only God can forgive guilt (ebenda, Theses 5 and 7). The Church can only proclaim this forgiveness, or the Church can forgive only punishments ordered by the Church discipline.

According to Luther, penance has only two parts: contrition (contritio) and trust (fides) to the words proclaiming the forgiveness of sins and the remission of guilt (without satisfaction). The "sola fide" of Reformation theology implied a deepened concern for sin and a vivid and honest feeling of guilt.

While medieval theology placed greater emphasis on act-sins (peccata actualia), Protestant theology emphasized the original/hereditary sin (peccatum originale).[9] Subsequently the

---

9 Original sin as a potential of sin realizes in the act of sin (peccatum actuale). Only the act of sin brings about guilt. Cf. Carson, 2002, 148–156. See as well:

teaching of sin was radicalized both by Lutheran and Calvinist theologians (Allen, 2010, 95-107). Relevant is Luther's definition of the true subject matter of theology in his extensive lecture on Psalm Miserere (Ps 51). The proper subject of all theology is: "man guilty of sin and condemned God his Justifier and Savior of man the sinner" ("ut proprie sit subiectum Theologiae homo reus et perditus et deus iustificans vel salvator"), with an addendum: "[W]hatever is asked or discussed in theology outside of this subject, is error and poison" (LW 12, 311). Guilt arises from the violation of trust in God as the absence of faith. According to a great expert on Lutheran Theology, E. Kinder: "In any case, man is essentially determined by the relationship with God How I fundamentally feel about God is how I fundamentally am. Justitia ... consists in the fact that one's existence is completely aligned (adjusted) towards God. ... Every sin is in principle a sin against the first Commandment" (Kinder, 1959, 40-41). In relation to people, it is an egoistic distortion of a person into himself as an absence of love (Batka, 2014). The whole weight of guilt was laid on the original sin. The problem of this concept rests in the fact that the guilt of original sin becomes universal doom of every human, creating a predicament of guilt (homo reatus et perditus).[10] We observed this conjunction of the sin, guilt, and punishment in the Hebrew Language and the Greek term "hamartia". E. Kinder summarizes: "Here what God's wrath condemns man for and what it punishes him with are identical. God punishes sin, which remains originally and fundamentally culpable, with the compulsion to sin. Culpa and poena – guilt and punishment – are rolled into one here" (Kinder, 1959, 66). Guilt and the tragical consequence of sin cannot be separated: "In every concrete act of sin or individual sin of mind, the culpable original sin and the fateful original sin

---

"Scholastic theologians say that original sin (concupiscentia) is only the ... 'conditio peccati' (condition for sin), 'fomes peccati' ('tinder' for sin), or on the other hand 'poena peccati' (punishment for sin), etc., but not itself sin in the full sense" (Kinder, 1959, 62).

10 It is beyond the scope of this article, but is should be pointed to the juridical interpretations of the guilt of original sin. According to Anselm of Canterbury, this kind of guilt cannot be done away because even if a person would obey God from today on, the guilt of not trusting him yesterday would remain. Thus, the question of atonement and satisfaction became relevant and had its influence up into the era of Reformation.

are expressed at the same time, and both manifest themselves anew together" (Kinder, 1959, 72).

Similarly to the Hebrew understanding of sin, the guilt arises from the violation of man's relationship with God. It originates in the heart of man; therefore, the salvation from sin is the transformation of the heart (Ps 51, 12, Mt 15, 19-20, cf. Mt 7, 17-20) and justification. The violation of this relationships creates guilt. The wrongdoing can be generally circumscribed as absent love for another person (Sum of the Law, Mt 22, 38-40).

In the development of Protestant churches, a similar practical question arose as before in medieval time, how to raise a sincere contrition in human heart? While medieval sacrament of penance the regret over a sinful act was emphasized, in Reformation theology a feeling of guilt about the condition of sin played a greater role. Instead of confessing "mea culpa", the Protestant confess "I am totally a sinner". The emphasis shifted to the inner man, to the subjective feeling in the heart and in the conscience. This problem led to the development of pietism of late 17th and 18th century, when the intensity of feeling of guilt (and of being forgiven and loved by God) should overcome the neo-scholastic doctrinal theology of protestant orthodoxy (Hausamann, 1974, 241-269). The practice of piety was rooted in inner experience and was expected to express in a life of religious commitment. This movement vehemently - again and again up to the present time - heightens the experience of guilt and fear (Künkler, Faix Jäckel, 2020).

Guilt Inside of Conscience and Feeling

Friedrich Schleiermacher represents a subjectivistic conception of guilt that exists only in the self-conscious mind. The consciousness of sin is connected exclusively with the awareness of oneself as dependent on the consciousness of God. As soon as human condition is spoken about as sinful, God consciousness is there. It is the basic framework in which the consciousness of sin can and must develop (Cf Axt-Piscalar, 1996, 231-237, Dalferth, 2020, 209).

The roots of his strong emphasis on feeling as the basis of religion rest in the religious upbringing of the revival movement from Herrnhut. His reinterpretation is admirably consistent, however at the cost of breaking away from theology of the reformers in many respects. Schleiermacher accepted the Christian teaching on sin and guilt, but fundamentally transformed it in accordance with his theological presuppositions. He wanted to avoid the Manichean position (evil nature) on one side and the Pelagianism (denial of original sin) on the other. However, the Augustinian solution about a humanity as massa damnata under a hereditary guilt (Erbschuld) was equally not satisfying to him. The importance of his contribution rest in thinking about original sin and guilt beyond the limits of rationalistic morality.

In his major work "*The Christian Faith*" ("*Der christliche Glaube*" (GL), 1821/22), Schleiermacher followed up on his theory of religion from the 2nd edition of his treatise "*Religion. Speeches to Its Cultured Despisers*" ("Über *die Religion. Reden an die Gebildeten unter ihren Verächtern*", 1799). Faith is not a matter of reason, but of feeling (in the 1st edition of "*Religio*", he spoke about *Anschauung*/intuition). By religiosity, Schleiermacher means a certain immediate feeling of dependence on God, that God lives and works in us as finite human beings. This feeling appears in a person's consciousness before rational reflection, an "original act of the spirit before the differentiation of the spirit in thinking, feeling and willing, but especially a process of self-consciousness that does not recognize the division into subject and object, as carried out by objective cognition" (Schleiermacher, 1999, XXXI).

For this article, especially relevant are the §70–74 of his "The Christian Faith". (A detailed analysis of this section offers Axt-Piscalar (Axt-Piscalar, 1996, 236–282).

The feeling of absolute dependence on God means consciousness (Bewusstsein) of oneself as a person living in an already predetermined relationship with God. It is an immediate relationship. A pure feeling of this absolute dependence on God represents the life and person of Jesus Christ. In any other person, these pious moments of feeling of absolute dependence on God do not appear with such direct conscience. They are clouded and inhibited, so everyone needs salvation. Sin is "having forgotten God" (Gottvergessenheit). However, it never appears in an absolute form (GL §11.2, 77). The consciousness of God can always be revived.

According to Schleiermacher, sin depends on the consciousness of God. Therefore, it cannot rest in the nature of man (GL §72, Leitsatz. GL §72.3, 386). It is not possible to talk about sin as an object of knowledge. It is always only self-conscience.[11] For this reason, "Adam's fall into sin" (peccatum originale) cannot be a historical event in Schleiermacher's system – which can be considered as a strong point of his argument. One cannot even speak of a state of "loss of natural perfection" in men or in humanity. Regarding the teaching of so-called "hereditary sin", two questions arise for Schleiermacher: How is it possible to "inherit" sinfulness and how can someone's sin cause another person´s personal guilt?

For this article, the second question is especially relevant: How can "hereditary" guilt be credited to a person? Original sin is a potentiality (Anlage), which becomes an ability (Fähigkeit) through a deed, and this then continues to grow (GL §71.1, 375). In the main sentence of paragraph GL §71, Schleiermacher says: "Inherited sin is at the same time the fault of every single person who has a share in the sin, so it can best be imagined as a totality of deeds and the total fault of the human race" (GL §71. Leitsatz, 374). We recognize this when we recognize the universal dependency for salvation.

Hereditary sin can be marked as guilt (reatus) only if: "[I]t is perceived as a collective deed of the entire generation" (GL §71.2, 378). It is not someone else's guilt (e.g. Adam) nor can we talk about punishment for someone else's sin (like in Augustine's masa perditionis). It is not the addition of Adam's guilt, but a guilt that is the same as Adam's. Everyone is responsible for the guilt. The contradiction of "hereditary sin" and "personal guilt" is solved by Schleiermacher as follows: since sin does not appear in a person without a personal individual will and since sin would arise through (each) person, it is possible to speak of the guilt of original sin (GL §71.1, 376). Hereditary sin brings guilt (even in children) only in the overall context (Zusammenhang) in which it is considered.

---

11 Cf. the title of GL §66: Explanation of sin as self-consciousness. Erklärung der Sünde als Selbstbewußtsein.

Equal and common guilt exists for all, but unlike the original guilt of Adam, which would be "inherited" to the next generations, it is a common and total guilt of humanity (GL §72.6, 397–398). Transmission of sin (and guilt) cannot take place in body (by procreation, sexuality). Sin is transmitted in education and cultural aspects of individual historical epochs. Even "inherited guilt" (Erbschuld) does not exist in itself, but as a cultural "inherited" doom ("Erb"-Verhängnis). No person can escape it, since everybody receives and accepts (mitempfängt und mitbekommt) not only his good but also his bad sides (GL §69.1, 366).

In the state of sinfulness, a person experiences in her consciousness (Selbstbewußtsein) the consciousness of guilt and the feeling of being worthy of a punishment. However, in turning to the consciousness of communion in life with Christ, a God-oriented consciousness is more strongly formed, thereby reducing the consciousness of guilt and of a feeling of being worthy of a punishment. In a system that is consistently based on the principle of active awareness of phenomena, conscience is a space that either prophetically warns against action or subsequently accompanies a person as an internal reproach, which can be followed by a feeling of guilt (GL §66.1, 356). If there is consciousness of sin, there is also conscience of God. Conscience is "the requirement of inward conformity with the consciousness of God within us" and regret is "holding on in the consciousness of what has passed away" (GL §108.2, 157). True remorse is a reflexively internalized consciousness.

According to Schleiermacher, the starting point is individual human being. His existence constantly alternates between remaining within himself and stepping out. Sin, guilt, and remorse are a constant, dynamic, pluralistic, and multifaceted process of change. Each belongs to this process and is not objectively opposed to it. Therefore, a person does not perceive it cognitively as a place of knowledge, nor voluntaristically as a place of action. A person experiences it in its originality with the feelings of "Lust" and "Unlust". Schleiermacher offers a psychological understanding of guilt. Guilt is a passive feeling: I am touched, taken, and moved by it. Guilt is related to self-conscience and self-judgment. Since there is a feeling of absolute dependence on God, there must be a feeling of guilt. But, in case the consciousness of God is abolished, there would not be guilt at all. This conclusion is elaborated with all sharpness in well-known Friedrich Nietzsche.

Annihilation of Guilt

Nietzsche's radical polemic against objective guilt and subjective feelings of guilt aims at Kantian universal "you shall" and rational reinterpretation of "conscience" as forum internum (Kant) – even more so at Christian radical interpretation of guilt.

In his most provocative and influential work "*On the Genealogy of Morals*" (1887), Nietzsche rewrote the history of ethics. His main question was: "Under what conditions did man invent the value-judgments good and evil?" (Nietzsche, 1996, 5). The original ethics of the strong ones (the will of life, courage, confidence) became replaced by the ethics of slaves. The weak ones promoted compassion, equality, and justice: "the inexorable progress of the morality of compassion, which afflicted even the philosophers with its illness, as the most sinister [*unheimlich*] symptom of the sinister development of our European culture" (ebenda, 7). History of ethics is a regress in – what is today perceived as – "moral", respectively, "good person". (Nietzsche opposed Darwin's view of evolution of humanity as a growth into morality.) The strong and superior "were the ones who felt themselves and their actions to be good – that is, as of the first rank – and presented them as such, in contrast to everything low, low-minded, common, and plebeian" (ebenda, 12). Originally, "good" was not identical with "unegoistic". This development is a regress of the "herd-instinct" and a sort of "mental illness" leading to an opposition to what was originally meant as good by the aristocratic superiors (ebenda, 13).

Fatal role in the process of transformation played the priests with their spiritual concept of hierarchy who turned away from (strong, free, high-spirited) actions to emotional volatility: "With the priests, everything becomes more dangerous, not only cures and therapies, but also arrogance, revenge, astuteness, extravagance, love, the desire to dominate, virtue, illness" (ebenda, 18). According to Nietzsche, Zoroaster was the first to introduce into religion the dualism of "good" and "evil", "immanence" and "transcendence". Judaism (the religion of priests), Christianity, Platonism "transvaluated" the good, noble, powerful, beautiful, happy, and blessed into the low, miserable, poor, powerless, the suffering, sick, ugly, and deprived (ebenda, 19). Symbolically, the "Tree of Knowledge of good and evil" became – according to Nietzsche – "the tree of revenge and hatred", that brought forth the "new love" (love toward the other) as a sign of hatred to all former noble ideals ("we the noble", "we the good", "we the beautiful", and "we the happy ones"). The slave, man of ressentiment, perceives himself as "good" and his enemies as "evil" people. In Nietzsche´s first essay, the distinction between "bad" and "evil" is crucial. Whereas "bad" is an original notion of noble aristocratic people, who took their point as spontaneously as "good", "evil" is a creation of slave morality speaking about the "noble, powerful, dominating man" as evil (ebenda, 25). "Ressentiment operates primarily in the mode of retroactivity, positing its derived values as original, once the aristocratic values on the nobility have been discredited through the slave revolt in morals" (ebenda, 48).

First developed the religion, than the culture, breeding "a tame and civilized animal, a domestic animal" (ebenda, 27). It is displayed in unnatural avoidance of the drive, will, and action and in demands "of strength that it should not express itself as strength, that it should not be a will to overcome, overthrow, dominate, a thirst for enemies and resistance and triumph" (ebenda, 29). If we stop here for a while and think about the consequences of Nitzschean de-transformation of concepts, the guilt arises as a non-complemency with those (unnatural) demands. Nietzsche radically rejects the Christian "masterpiece of black magic" to proclaim the refusal of revenge as justice "we good men – we are the just" (ebenda, 32) According to Nietzsche, ethical norms are a slave revolt against the aristocratic morality of hegemony.

In the second essay in *"On the Genealogy of Morals"* related to guilt and bad conscience, Nietzsche develops his arguments about the active nobility in a more general – and for his thinking central – notion of "will to power": "The essence of life, ..., the priority of the spontaneous, attacking, overcoming, reinterpreting, restructuring and shaping forces" (ebenda, 59). This will of power sets upon the less powerful and impresses the meaning of concepts (like promise, punishment, debt, guilt) upon the subjugated in accordance with its own interests. In the earliest contractual relations between individuals arose the notion of "debt" (Schulden, dlh). The promise of repayment was made and in order "to impress repayment as a duty and obligation sharply at his conscience, the debtor contractually pledges to the creditor in the event on non-payment something ... over which he still has power" (ebenda, 45). This resembles the political contract theory. However, Nietzsche concentrates on the inequality and power relation between debtor and creditor, which includes the right to inflict punishment and pain "the most powerful aid to memory" (ebenda, 43). The contract became the vehicle for the active strong to impose their will to power. The debt gave them the right to inflict punishment, in case the debtor became guilty (schuldig) in not repaying the debt to the creditor. Nietzsche is the legal obligation prior to the moral conception of guilt and duty and personal responsibility. Guilt is connected to the threat of pain so that a person does not forget its promises and the creditor gets gratified through the suffering in the punishment of the debtor.

On a societal level, the wrongdoing of breaking (brechen) of contractual commitment to society (of breaking ones word of the promise) makes a person a "Verbrecher" (criminal) losing the access to the goods and advantages of the whole community (ebenda, 52); thus, all societal development and law are a product of economically sanctioned violence.

In this regard, Nietzsche's interpretation of the origin of law is interesting. It is not surprising that the law is seen as a process of the stronger, nobler, braver, and more aggressive man to get revenge and to compel a settlement between the weaker parties: "Whenever justice is practiced, whenever justice is upheld, one sees a stronger power seeking means to put an end to the senseless ragging of ressentiment among the weaker powers subordinate to it" (ebenda, 56). In a positivist manner, Nietzsche argues that the strong sets the principles of right and wrong and that there is nothing essentially wrong in violation, destruction (will of power). In other words, on the side of the wrong and active ones, there is only (free) conscience. The notion of "bad conscience" is the invention of the man of ressentiment, subjugated to the more powerful active noble man. Nevertheless, the love of freedom – i.e.

the will to power – turns inward and in the process of internalization, man turns against himself. All hostility, cruelty, and pleasure in persecution, assault, and destruction are channeled to the feeling of "bad conscience". For Nietzsche this state is nothing less as a "sinister sickness" as the will to "mistreat the self" (ebenda, 67-68) and to self-torture "in order to inflict pain on himself after the more natural outlet for his desire to inflict pain was obstructed" (ebenda, 72).

Not surprisingly the moralization of the concept of debt and duty happened in the realm of religion. Human debt against God gets its radical and inhuman extent in notions of redeemability of guilt, insufficiency of penance, and impossibility of repayment creating a religious bad conscience in its ultimate and horrific dimensions. Religion is madness of the will in psychic cruelty and the only cure for man is atheism, the realm of "second innocence", a radical antichristian, and antinihilist attitude (Antichrist) seeking new liberty through Zarahrustra the godless (ebenda, 72-76). Bad conscience disappears as soon as the repression of the active instincts and turning toward oneself stops. In this perception the human history is not a progress toward greater equality and compassion but a history of cruelty, imposed socially (state and law) and self-inflicted (morality and religion).

Nietzsche's approach is valuable in his conceptual and etymological analysis of the terminology related to good and bad, good and evil, or guilt. He pointed out several important connections between guilt and pain, and prepared the soil for a Freudian analysis of conscience and the violent character of repression. Nietzsche attempted to show true origins of moral concepts. argued that moral values and guilt are contingent products of historical struggle; they are derived from material basis (economy of credit and debt); and finally, the guilt and bad conscience are pathologized in psychological structures and processes. Religion convinces the weak that they are responsible for their own suffering.

Both Schleiermacher and Nietzsche – though in opposite ways – understand that the will operates in structures that are given. Both think that the "evil" structures are result of human actions (whereas Nietzsche seems the religious actions as particularly "perverse".) This means, human will is not itself a matter of the will´s choice. While I am who I am through my willing, my willing is shaped by a fundamental condition in every concrete act. Both thinkers struggled with structures of guilt that define the existence of man. A half century later offered a hermeneutics of Dasein, that brought a new perspective on the guilt.

The Guilty Existence of Man

In *Being and Time* (1927), Martin Heidegger explores the concept of guilt (*Schuld*) within the broader context of his existential analysis of human existence (*Da-sein*). The psychological, biological, and theological explanations are not sufficient for his inquiry. In §54-§60 he analyzed conscience phenomenologically (first-person perspective), focusing on the experience from the perspective of Dasein (hermeneutics of Da-sein). The primordial phenomenon of *Da-sein* which is in everyday interpretation of itself presents to us as the "voice of conscience". Conscience is an inner call, not present as a fact rather as a (silent) voice. The call of conscience discloses existential guilt and urges authentic existence (Heidegger 1996, 249). The call of conscience summons "the self to its potentiality-of-being-a-self, and thus calls Dasein forth to its possibilities." (ebenda, 253). The meaning is to get out from the absorption of man in the everyday, inauthentic mode of existence to its own most potentiality-for-being, since "it is a Da-sein in its uncanniness, primordially thrown being-in-the-world, as not-at-home, the naked "that" in the nothingness of the world." (ebenda, 255). Uncanniness in everyday life is not conscious, but for Heidegger, it is the fundamental way of being in the world. Conscience is an "attestation" in Da-sein of its own most potentiality-of-being (§57). The call of conscience "directs Da-sein forward toward its potentiality-of-being, as a call out of uncanniness" (ebenda, 258).

Conscience has a temporal structure and points to the finite existence and to the impossibility of fulfilling all potentialities of man. Since in the experience, the conscience is related to guilt (as already guilty, possibility of becoming guilty, or not being guilty in good conscience), in §58 Heidegger went on to analyze the calling in relation to guilt. For our text is central his question how people are guilty and what guilt means?

The basic meaning of German "*Schuldigsein*" is of "owing something", "having something on account", "having debts". Further related notions are depriving, borrowing, withholding, taking, and robbing. But they all are related to things that can be acquired. Second significance is related to cause. Being the author or causa of something. This second kind of guilt is not related to things. A person can be guilty (*Schuld haben an*) without "owing" anything to someone else (ebenda, 260). Third kind of guilt is related to the law, in the significance of "becoming responsible to others". This kind of responsibility is related to solidarity. The guilt means "a lacking and it is a failure to satisfy some demand placed on one's existing being-with others" (ebenda, 260). Similar to it is Jaspers "metaphysical guilt", but Heidegger calls it a "moral guilt". Moral guilt arises from specific actions or omissions that violate ethical or legal norms. In contrast, existential guilt is more fundamental and is tied to the very nature of Dasein's being.

Heidegger's aim is to go deeper to the idea of guilt in terms of the kind of being of Da-sein. It must be some kind of fundamental "primordial being guilty". From the inherent limitations and finitude of human life, laying behind the possibilities into which the Da-sein is thrown, not being able to gain power over the very ownmost being shows a negativity ("not") of existential being guilty: "Da-sein as such is guilty" (ebenda, 263). Paradoxically, Da-sein is always guilty because it is thrown into a world where it must make choices and take responsibility for its existence, yet it cannot fulfill every potential or actualize all possibilities. "Being whose being is care can not only burden themselves with factual guilt, but they are guilty in the ground of their being" (ebenda, 264). Being guilty precedes the knowing about it. Conscience calls Da-sein to confront its own guilt and the limitations of its existence so that it can become more authentic. Authenticity involves acknowledging one's finitude and the inevitable shortcomings that come with being a finite, thrown being. This recognition leads Dasein to take ownership of its existence, it opens way to a genuine and moral life: "[T]he ownmost possibility that Da-sein can give itself as a calling back that calls it forth to its factical potentiality-of-being-a-self. To hear the call authentically means to bring oneself to factical action" (ebenda, 271). Heidegger connects this existential structure of guilt with the "mood" of anxiety (*Angst*). Anxiety and silence open space to confront the "nullity" of Da-sein, as well as one's mortality (being-towards-Death, cf. §§ 46–53) by "resoluteness". According to Heidegger, only authentic, resolute mode of existence is able to become open for its world, and other "beings". It takes care of them, and "discloses that potentiality in concern which leaps ahead and frees" (ebenda, 274). Without being-with-one-another, there is not possibility for being-with-one-another. For Nietzsche, the authentic self ends up in subjugating others. The "conscience" for the strong ones become the poor and weak, with theirs claims of solidarity and fraternity. For Heidegger the authentic self is able to respect the being of others, and to take care, without subjugation, stipulation or a "slavish identification with" (or a slavish differentiation from) others (Mulhall 2005, 146). Despite the existential guilt and inauthenticity, all humans are capable of living authentically, even though Heidegger does not give a clear explanation how this transition from within is possible (ebenda, 144).

A serious attempt to explain the importance of myths of fall into sin, and the symbols of sin and guilt represents the extensive work of French Philosopher Paul Ricoeur.

Symbol of Sin, Meaning of Guilt

Paul Ricœur sought to establish links between present day scholarship and the Jewish and Christian exegetical tradition. For our topis is especially relevant his phenomenology of religion. He applied his hermeneutical approach to the fundamental ethical dimension of sin and guilt and showed how religious experiences reflect on reality by using symbolical language. "Symbols make us think", they are an indirect expression of things that are holy for a person. (Ricoeur, 1974, vol ii., 258). The methodology of phenomenology leads to the wider understanding of the meaning of guilt and makes sensitive to the fact that human reason is not an autonomous entity, but is, so to speak, anchored in an existence that subdues human intentionality as desire and effort. Ricoeur looks at guilt from the perspective: what do I experience in the feeling of guilt as well as what does the symbol of sin reveal about us?

In his exceptionally subtle hermeneutical analysis of human existence, Ricoeur is aware that naturalism and especially psychoanalysis raise an important question about the "lie of consciousness" or even more profound, about the "consciousness as lie". In that case, the conscious feeling of guilt appears to be just a projection of a philosopher and needs to be "de-mythologized" by a psychiatric and psychoanalytic work. He dedicated his major work: "*The Fallible Man*" from 1971, to interpret the meaning of symbols of sin and to analyze the real structure of guilt.

Guilt can exist only because a person exists in relation to another person. Human self always exists between two. It is a transition between me and the other: "But an attempt must be made to grasp this difference of the self beyond the side of self-preference" (Ricoeur, 1971, vol. i., 142). Self-preference, rather than communion between two leads to hostile attitudes toward other people. This is where the space for guilt arises. The constitution of difference includes a structure of fallibility in self-preference. In this way, guilt becomes possible, but not inevitable.

Ricoeur describes the human experience as marked by a certain chronic disproportion, an incessant inner discord, because of which man can never come to an agreement with himself. This disproportion is shown in every aspect of human existence, from perception to feeling to thinking. It is visible, for example, in the human desire, even addiction (Sucht) for possessions, power, or prestige. Humans are by nature fragile and prone to making mistakes.

Ricoeur argues for the importance of feelings: "The general function of feeling is to create connection. It connects what knowledge divides. It binds me back to things, to beings, to being" (Ricoeur, 1971, vol. i., 171). Through reason I view the others as objects. In feelings, my intentionality and affects come together. Feelings bring me to "here and now", and in this way they overcome the subject-object split. Two intentions struggle in my feeling: intention of "happiness in every moment" and the intention of "desire for wholeness and perfection". The "mind" mediates between these two basic intentions. But it is not without conflicts. In the conflict of subjectivity, the feeling of guilt can develop (Ricoeur, 1971, vol. i., 172, Connection to Kant in Chappell, 2019, 230).

Man is fallible. This means that "the possibility of moral evil is written into the human condition" (Ricoeur, 1971, vol. i., 173). The fallibility rests in the weakness of human beings that becomes apparent in the complexity between (1) possibility and origin and (2) between origin and ability. Ricoeur accepts the scholastic Kantian notion of evil as "nihil privativum": "there is a gap, a leap, from this possibility to the reality of evil: therein lies the whole riddle of guilt" (Ricoeur, 1971, vol. i., 183).

In the first instance, fallibility means only the "possibility" of evil, the structure of reality, that makes space (a zone) for the origin of evil. For ethics, this implies that human beings are able of both: of the valuable and the non-valuable, of the true and false, of the beautiful and ugly.[12] In ethics, the task is to find a middle between two non-correct extremes. What makes Ricoeurs hermeneutical approach interesting is his conviction that in the realm of ethics, the human predicament is a starting point of fallibility: Ethics wants to educate, "raise" (erziehen), and build up from a realm that is already defined by fallibility (Ricoeur, 1971, vol. i., 185). Man already missed the goal and forgot its origins. "Since then, the puzzle has been the 'jump' from the fallible to the already fallen. Our anthropological reflection remained on this side of the leap, ... ethics started too late. To capture it, we must start from the beginning, to initiate a new reflection that considers the confession that consciousness makes about itself and that pursues the symbols of evil in which this confession is expressed" (ebenda, 185).

The second aspect speaks about the complexity between origin and ability, the possibility to evil. Noteworthy is Ricoeur's reflection of the predicament that makes possible the "transgression", "detour", "de-railing". The original can be recognized in the "evil" like behind a wail. "In this way, the evil of failure intentionally points to the original. Conversely, however, this reference to the original constitutes evil as a transgression" (ebenda, 187, Cf. ebenda, ch. 4, 140–163).

Is the "original state" a state of innocence? According to Ricoeur only in human imagination. A state of innocence is no place in geography and history. It is only an imagination of "somewhere else"

---

12 Concerning moral emotions and aesthetics cf. Kišoňová, 2023, Démuth, Démuthová, Keceli, 2023.

or "before" as expressed in myths. Ricoeur uses here the methodology of Husserl's eidetic imagination as modus of exploring the real one. "What is essential about the myth of innocence is that it provides a symbol of the original that shines through the depravity and shows it as depravity. My innocence is my original constitution, projected into a fantastic story" (ebenda, 187, 147).

Here, we can look briefly at the concept of *"Dreaming Innocence"* by P. Tillich. At first glance, Ricoeur´s position resembles Tillich´s. Tillich does not consider any state of ideal conditions before the fall to be necessary and adopts (Kierkegaard's) concept of "dreaming innocence", which precedes actual existence as a mere potentiality. Tillich psychologically described this situation using the example of sexuality in a person's life. Until a certain point in time, the child is completely unaware of his sexual potential (Tillich, 1967, 34). Similarly, it is with an adolescent who finds himself tempted to actualize his freedom by losing his "dreaming innocence" or chooses to preserve his innocence by having to deal with the anxiety of sacrificing his sexual possibilities. Dreaming Innocence is "dreaming" since it is not directly accessible to the waking state. It only appears there in a fragmented, distorted way like any dream. It is "innocent" because it lacks the "experience", "responsibility", and "guilt" that every actual event entails but nevertheless has them before it as a possibility. Tillich's identification of creation and fall, ontologized the historical (transition from essence to existence) and robbed it of moral significance.

The possibility of fallibility thus implies that before transgression there is a possibility of no-transgression. Even the transgression is something original, the non-transgression is even more original, or to express it with Ricoeur: "As original as evil may be, goodness is even more original" (ebenda, 188). We saw, that according to Heidegger, the existential guilt is not "transgression", rather an "omission" of possibilities. It resembles to the "fallibility" by Ricoeur, whereas for Ricoeur the failure points to the original, that is better. For Heidegger, the "not" is the "first" and the nullity is the fundament.

Ricoeur does not think that there was an historical period of "before the fall into sin", but in his interpretation of the symbol, he thinks that there is a possibility to think a better original. His ethical concern widens the perspective from one single deed to the ability and to the totality of life. Beyond duties and virtues his interest is to give meaning to the existence which can appear as one indivisible fate of "evil".

What than can be seen like through a wail on the background of transgression? Hate and war show the intersubjective structure of respect and responsibility. The misunderstanding and lie let shine through the identity and otherness in self-conscious. The obsession with having, exercising power, prestige (*Habsucht, Herrschsucht, Ehrsucht*) show the fundamental forms of existence of to have, to be able to, and to be respected. Here, Ricoeur accept Kant´s anthropological trilogy of passions. The obsession (*Sucht*) is like a "delirium", and so is their appearance in human history, as something that "went of the track". Similarly to Nietzsche, Ricoeur accepts the economical-historical analysis of the origin of personal property (and of work). Private ownership (economic sphere), exercise of authority (political sphere), and expectations of respect (sphere of self-consciousness) are not the source of evil. Power can be natural as a technological necessity to overcome the adversary condition of nature, or as economical-social institutions confirming the authority of the individuum, the group or state: "Authority is not inherently bad. Commanding is a necessary "differentiation" among people, inherent in the nature of politics" (ebenda, 153). Likewise, the wish to be respected among other people, the search for esteem itself are not negative.

In difference to Nietzsche, the revolt of the weak ones does not create the negative interpretation of will and power. According to Ricoeur, whereas the ownership of property is just, the passion "to have" can get out of hand in the obsession of greed, in passions of gluttony, stingy, and envy (ebenda, 148–149). Greed for power becomes a passion for commanding and using violence. Vanity and presumption pervert the esteem in greed for prestige (*Ehrsucht*). This third aspect touches the level of self-conscience; thus, its perversion implies the disturbance in interpersonal relations: "The self-esteem that I secure through the way of being valued by others is no different from the high regard that I feel for others. If it is humanity that I value in others and in myself, then I value myself as a you to others. I value myself in the second person" (ebenda, 162).

The fallibility means not only the possibility in weakness, but likewise the ability to transgress. The myths of fall in sin are for

Ricoeur meaningful instruments to speak about this transition. He compares it to a state of "dizziness", permanent transition in staggering, sliding over between fallibility and fall.

He has shown the usefulness of the symbol of "original sin" and its meaning. Like Protestant theology before Schleiermacher, Ricoeur understands the relational aspect of sin: "The basic symbolism of sin expresses the loss of a connection, a rootedness, an ontological ground" (Ricoeur, 1971, vol. ii., 85).

One of the most interesting parts of Ricoeurs phenological analysis is the conclusion about the reality of sin – moving behind Schleiermacher. The objective evil is the "heart of a person", his existence, no matter how aware he is of it (Ricoeur, 1971, vol. ii., 97). Here, originates Ricoeur´s talk about the "reality of sin". The second aspect of the reality of sin is its personal but likewise its communitarian aspect: "we the sinners". Confessions of sins happened in a community. The "we have sinned" makes sin an egalitarian concept. (The sin is, or is not: all are sinners, all committed some sinful act.) The symbol of "original sin" is a bad term because it tries to make the communitarian aspect by means of pseudo-biological and pseudo-juridical language rational (Ricoeur, 1960). The third aspect of the reality of sin is the theological perspective that every sin is a sin "in conspectu dei". From God´s point of view, every sin is a sin, regardless of what my conscience might say. Ricoeur came close to the Protestant interpretation of sin. For him it represents the "structural continuity" that acts as a "power" toward "alienation" and "adulteration" (Ricoeur, 1971, vol. ii., 102–107).

Ricoeur saw the tension between the "realism" of sin and the "phenomenalism" of the feeling of guilt. In the consciousness of wrongdoing, according to the scheme of sin, "evil" is a situation "inside" humanity trapped as a collective of its own kind. According to the guilt "evil" is an act done by each person individually (Ricoeur, 1971, vol. ii., 124).

Guilt is personal and individual. It is an "I" who is guilty. In law, criminal law, but in ethics too, one can be more guilty, another less guilty (Ricoeur, 1974, vol. ii., 271). The personalization and individualization lead to the question of the consciousness of guilt.

The Feeling of Guilt

There is a difference between being guilty and feeling guilty. The question about guilt as emotion or a feeling rest in the difference in apprehension of the subjective or objective aspect of guilt. The book *"The Moral Psychology of Guilt"* (Cokelet, Maley, 2019, 11–110) offers vivid discussion on this question. Scholars such as C. Maley and G. Harman argue that guilt is not an emotion and regard it as a feeling. Guilt is a feeling about being guilty and that "there is no single emotion that is guilt. Some occurrences of feeling guilty might involve anxiety, other might involve anger, and still other might involve sadness" (Maley, Harman, 2019, 28). According to them, in difference to emotions, feeling have a cognitive element and are more complex states.

To the extent that guilt becomes individualized, it acquires gradations. The egalitarian aspect of the experience of sin is opposed to the gradual aspect of the experience of guilt. According to Ricoeur, there is a double aspect in the feeling of guilt: "The feeling of guilt can be seen as an internalization and personalization of the consciousness of sin" (Ricoeur, 1971, vol. ii., 76).

By semantic analysis of guilt we can differentiate several categories (Ricoeur, 1974, vol. ii., 268–269):

1. of space: to miss the goal, to be lost, to wander around, to be like sand in the wind.

2. of intensity: to burn, to annihilate, to be empty, to be hollow, to burden, crush.

3. of disobedience: to be stubborn, rebellious, to lack faithfulness, to be adulterous.

4. of purity: blemish, impurity, stain, to get dirty.

5. of health: to be infected, to spread, to weaken, to make sick, to be eaten up (bites of conscience).

Conscience is a complex psycho-ethical framework related to empathy, self-scrutiny, and a change of attitudes. According to J. Cottingham, conscience, guilt (and shame) are primarily concerned with "the interior dimension of morality: how each of us thinks and feels about our own conduct when we review it, or when we measure it against our sense of what is expected of us, or how we might have done better" (Cottingham, 2013, 729).

Categories of space or disobedience bear cognitive aspect, and categories of intensity or purity bear predominantly emotional aspect. Under the rational cognitive aspect, such conscious self-observation, self-accusation, and self-condemnation resembles to a courtyard. To express it with I. Kant, the conscience resembles to "forum internum". In the second chapter of his *"The Metaphysic of Morals"* (1797), Kant replaced the heteronomous divine lawgiver with an autonomous lawgiver in the reason of man. Guilt and the accusing conscience (no longer the voice of God) represent the voice of practical reason. Conscience is normative in prescribing right and wrong before an action is done, or making a judgment about wrongdoing afterwards. This tribunal of reason is like a creation of "an ideal person that reason creates for itself", since nobody can be his or hers own judge. (Cottingham, 2013, 739, Chappell, 2019, 232).

The emotional aspect gets more accentuated in empirical, respectively, naturalist position. Guilt as psychological event is not normative since feelings are subjective. Painful sanctions of the feeling of guilt are not normative reasons for actions, rather reinforcement and inducement of compliance. (f.E. J.S. Mill).

S. Freud (Cf. *Totem and Taboo,* 1913) not only rejected the theistic view of the origins of conscience. According to him, conscience originates not in the "ego", but acts as an independent agency of the "super ego" (Over-I). The ambivalence between the unconscious desire and the conscious prohibition creates the feeling of guilt. Since the super-ego is not directly accessible to consciousness, the super-ego can drive to an aggressive cycle of self-criticism and demands of perfection. Freud speaks about the experience of guilt but is skeptical about its positive role. Guilt is rather an illness. Christian rituals are in effect an extended and collective form of guilt, based on the ancient forms of totemism and tabu. (Scharfenberg, 1969, 141–145).

The first explicit occurrence of a concept of conscience can be found in the *"Letter to Romans"* by Apostle Paul in New Testament. The passage reads: "They show that the work of the law is written on their hearts, while their conscience also bears witness, and their conflicting thoughts accuse or even excuse them" (R 2, 15). The Greek word "syneidesis" (συνείδησις), like the Latin term "conscientia" (Slovak: svedomie), expresses the idea of not being unconscious, present in the mind, but part of consciousness. According to Paul, the non-Jews (Romans and other nations), who did not know the Torah are able to recognize the principles of law written by nature in their syneidesis. Through a misspelling of the New Testament Greek the patristic writers start to speak about "synderesis" as a "spark of conscience", some innate God given disposition of "rational power" which enables to know right and wrong (Cottingham, 2013, 732, Chappell, 2019, 230-231, Baylor, 1977).

As we have seen by the notion of sin, the Hebrew thinking is holistic. It does not set the rational against the emotional. The Hebrew term עָדִי (jadá) means "to know" (ginóskó in Greek), to ascertain by seeing (corresponding to the Greek eidon – to see, similarly to Slovak vedieť and vidieť). It has as well the experiential part of knowledge: to perceive, to acquire knowledge, to know, to be acquainted. It can be used in a great variety of senses, including observation, care, and recognition. This can be applied to sense of touch but likewise to the hearth or mind. That which results from seeing, experience is a sort of understanding. Thus, the term can imply to feel, or to care as well. Often it is used as a euphemism for sexual intercourse. The Biblical "Tree of Knowledge of good and evil" in Paradise (Gen 2,17) is not a tree of artificial intelligence. The human intelligence encompasses knowledge, experience, and feelings.

The Biblical story of the Prophet Nathan confronting King David (2 Sam 12, 1-15) offers a powerful narrative showing the feeling of guilt. In this story, God sends Nathan, a trusted prophet, to confront David about his sin. Uriah was buried and Bathsheba was nine months pregnant. Nathan uses a parable of a rich man who unjustly takes a poor man's beloved lamb to illustrate David's own transgression. By the narrative story, Nathan touches on David's feelings and empathy. The words of Nathan direct David inwards to a disapproval felt by transgression of another person. David's response to the parable, where he passionately condemns the rich man's actions, sets the stage for Nathan's revelatory statement, "You are the man!" This direct confrontation shatters David´s blindness and brings him face to face with the gravity of his own wrongdoings. David came face to face with his own sin and his immediate response was a feeling of guilt and confession of guilt: "I have sinned against the Lord." (This exemplifies genuine repentance – acknowledging the offense, taking responsibility, and turning back to God.) He acknowledged his guilt, and it became known to him. In the Church tradition Psalm 51 was regarded as David's confession of guilt: "Against you, you alone, have I sinned and done what is evil in your sight, …" (Ps 51, 4) and "The sacrifice acceptable to God is a broken spirit; a broken and contrite heart, O God, you will not despise" (Ps 51, 17). "Once certain emotional and cognitive barriers are lifted, it is David's own conscience that convicts him" (Cottingham, 2013, 731). Besides the religious aspect of the story (sin toward God) and the theological recognition that by wrongdoing to another person the relationship to God is touched, there is an emotional aspect of the story: touching the empathy of a person. Ricoeur was able to see this holistic understanding of guilt: "The elevation of consciousness to conscience as the highest authority can be clearly seen in the feeling of guilt" (Ricoeur, 1971, vol. ii., 92).

Feeling of guilt implies an internal mental awareness of guilt at wrongdoing, related to certain situations in life, which is the the meaning of the word "conscientia". Likewise, the feeling of guilt torments a person as a burning feeling; in confessions of guilt, emotions of anger, fear, and sorrow are dominant.

Finally, we return to the question if guilt is useful for human society. The answer was that it is, but indirectly. The usefulness of guilt rests outside of the guilt. Guilt exists between persons (or a normative system preserving relations of persons). That means, guilt has its meaning when it prevents a wrongdoing or leads to a change in interpersonal relations.

The Greek term "metanoía" μετανοία means "change one´s mind", to alter the entire vision upon reality, to see reality in a new light (it appears over 55 times in New Testament). Thus, it is not only an intellectual or a psychological state but a relational and an existential act as well (Neumann, 2017, 42–46). In Hebrew, the reversal/turning around (בוּשׁ, šúb) is related to the image of a crooked way of going astray (expressions of sin). Turning around ends up in healing, salvation, and freedom (Ricoeur, 1971, vol. ii., 92). The full meaning of guilt (and sin) is understood from the point of view of "forgiveness". The feeling of guilt effects a change of perception, attitude, and behavior, and brings about a new start. The symbol of "delusion" seems suitable with its negative, pessimistic, and tragical influence on human acting. Through guilt, resistance, and by being blind, one is unable to recognize and feel the situation, and thus alienation, slavery, and captivation become part of human experience. Feeling guilt wakes up from delusion and dizziness in human conduct.

Conclusion

We avoided Ricoeur´s "conflict of interpretations" and spoke about guilt in net of interpretations. We have seen that the notion of guilt unites several traditions: the Greek-philosophical, the Roman-legal, and Biblical-religious. Despite differences, they are intertwined in several aspects.

We spoke about persons in a web of guilt. It means that nobody lives for itself. In this world people live in relationships, aspire ownership, power, and prestige. These are at first morally neutral natural dispositions. Naturally, people are fallible. In their pursuit, they become entangled in inclinations, they knot things by wrongdoing, and they are trapped in structures propagating "sin". The conflictedness of freedom and predicament becomes apparent in conscience. Sin, guilt, and punishment are at times hard to distinguish.

There is an ambivalence in guilt. It can be a safety net for responsible life according to moral ideals and legal norms. The feeling of guilt is a psychological support keeping people from violating relationships. It helps to preserve integrity on a personal level and responsibility on an intrapersonal level. A sensitive conscience reacts not only to transgressions but also avoids wrongdoing. Feeling of guilt is an indication of the value of relationships. The feeling of guilt opens the way to metanoia that means processes of healing, progress, and improvement.

On the opposite side, a too sensitive conscience strives for perfection. It leads to pedantry and legalism. An endless circle of self-observation, self-accusation, and self-condemnation becomes pathological and ends up in self-harm and self-inflicted pain. The condemnation turns to damnation. An overexaggerated feeling of guilt is pathological and harmful. Distortions of pathological (self) destruction and (self)harm are to be avoided. A healthy self-image includes conscience, but a conscience need not be guilty conscience all the time.

The fact of net interpretations of guilt shows that the growth of human culture, religiosity, philosophy, law, and complexity of social structures is related to the notion of guilt. Schleiermacher points to the inwardness of guilt in the conscience. Nietzsche repudiated guilt as something alien and external. Ricoeur has argued that sin is the real situation of man before God, and to be guilty is to become conscious about this real situation. Nevertheless, the negative symbol of sin shows something which is more original: the intersubjective structure of respect and responsibility.

References

Allen, R.M. (2010). *Reformed Theology*. T&T Clark.

Althaus, P. (1963). *Paulus und Luther* über *den Menschen. Ein Vergleich*. 4th ed. Gerd Mohn.

Aquinas, T. (1989). *Summa Theologiae. A Concise Translation* (STh). Ed. T. McDermott. Christian Classics.

Axt-Piscalar,Ch. (1996). *Ohnmächtige Freiheit. Studien zum Verhältnis von Subjektivität und Sünde bei August Tholuck, Julius Müller, Sören Kierkegaard und Friedrich Schleiermacher*. Mohr-Siebeck.

Batka, L. (2014). Luther's Teaching on Sin and Evil. In: R. Kolb, I. Dingel, & L. Batka (eds.). *The Oxford Handbook of Martin Luther's Theology*. Oxford University Press (pp. 233–253).

Batka, L. (2023). Spiritual and Theological Discernment of Good and Evil. In A. Démuth & S. Démuthová (eds.). *A Conceptual and Semantic Analysis of the Qualitative Domains of Aesthetic and Moral Emotions*. Peter Lang (pp. 101–118).

Baylor, M. (1977). *Conscience in Late Scholasticism and the Young Luther*. E. J. Brill.

Bauer, W. (1971). *Griechisch-Deutsches Wörterbuch zu den Schriften des Neuen Testaments und der übrigen urchristlichen Literatur*. 5. ed. De Gruyter.

Carson, T. (2002). *New Catholic Encyclopedia*. Vol 13. 2nd ed. Gate Research (pp. 148–156).

Chappell, S.-G. (2019). Conscience and Guilt from St. Paul to Nietzsche. In B. Cokelet & C. J. Maley (eds.).. *The Moral Psychology of Guilt*. Rowman & Littlefield (pp. 227–242).

Choe SY, Min K-H. (2011). Who Makes Utilitarian Judgments? The Influences of Emotions on Utilitarian Judgments. *Judgment and Decision Making*. 6(7), 580–592. doi:10.1017/S193029750000262X

Cottingham, J. (2013). Conscience, Guilt and Shame. In: R. Crisp. *The Oxford Handbook of the History of Ethics*. Oxford University Press (pp. 729–743).

Cross, F. L. (1997). *The Oxford Dictionary of the Christian Church*. Oxford University Press.

Crüsemann, F. (1992). "... wie wir vergeben unseren Schuldigern". Schulden und Schuld in der biblischen Tradition. In: M. Crüsemann & W. Schottroff (eds.). *Schuld und Schulden. Biblische Traditionen in gegenwärtigen Konflikten*. Chr. Kaiser (90–103).

Dalferth, I. (2020). *Sünde. Die Entdeckung der Menschlichkeit*. Evangelische Verlagsanstalt.

Démuth, A, Démuthová, S. Keceli, Y. (2023). On Some Etymological, Grammatical and Contextual Reasons for the Vagueness of the Concept of Beauty. In A. Démuth & S. Démuthová. *A Conceptual and Semantic Analysis of the Qualitative Domains of Aesthetic and Moral Emotions*. Peter Lang (p. 39–56).

De Hooge, I.E. (2019). Improving Our Understanding of Guilt by Focusing on Its (Inter)Personal Consequences. In B. Cokelet & C. J. Maley. *The Moral Psychology of Guilt*. Rowman & Littlefield (pp. 131–147).

Hausamann, S. (1974). *Buße als Umkehr und Erneuerung von Mensch und Gesellschaft*. Theologischer Verlag Zürich.

Heidegger, M. (1996). *Being and Time. A Translation of Sein und Zeit*. Transl. J. Stambaugh. State University of New York.

Jaspers, K. (2000). *The Question of German Guilt*. Fordham University Press.

Jenson, M. (2006). *The Gravity of Sin*. Bloomsbury Academics.

Kašný, J. (2017). *Právo v hebrejské Bibli*. Vyšehrad.

Kinder, E. (1959). *Die Erbsünde*. Schwabenverlag.

Kišoňová, R. (2023). Considering the Emotion of Disgust in the Context of Tešrminology and Contemporary Literature. In A. Démuth & S. Démuthová (eds.). *A Conceptual and Semantic Analysis of the Qualitative Domains of Aesthetic and Moral Emotions*. Peter Lang (pp. 81–100).

Knierim, R. (2001). Sünde. In ed. G. Müller (ed.). *Theologische Realenzyklopädie*, XXXII. De Gruyter (pp. 365–372).

Koch, R. (1992). *Die Sünde um Alten Testament*. Peter Lang.

Künkler, T., Faix, T., & Jäckel, M. (2020). The Guilt Phenomenon. An Analysis of Emotions towards God in Highly Religious Adolescents and Young Adults. In *Religions*. 11(8), 420. https://doi.org/10.3390/rel11080420

Luther's Works (LW), (1955). In J. Pelikan (ed.). Concordia Publishing House.

Maley, C. J., Harman, G. (2019). The Feeling of Guilt. In B. Cokelet & C.J. Maley (eds.). *The Moral Psychology of Guilt*. Rowman & Littlefield (pp. 12–36).

Meteňkanyč, O. (2023). The relevance of Legal Intuitionism and Selected Moral Emorions in Legal Thinking and Decision-Making Processes. In A. Démuth & S. Démuthová (eds.). *A Conceptual and Semantic Analysis of the Qualitative Domains of Aesthetic and Moral Emotions* (pp. 119-163). Peter Lang.

Moltmann, J. (1974). *Man: Christian Anthropology in the Conflicts of the Present*. S.P.C.K.

Mulhall, S. (2005). *Heidegger and Being and Time*. 2nd. ed. Routledge.

Neumann, N. (2017). Μετάνοια in neutestamentlichen Handlungsstrukturen. In: *Berliner Theologische Zeitschrift (BThZ), Buße* 34(1), 25-46.

Nietzsche, F. (1996). *On the Genealogy of Morals*. Oxford University Press.

Ohst, M. (1995). *Pflichtbeichte. Untersuchungen zum Bußwesen im Hohen und Späten Mittelalter*. Tübingen.

Panczová, H. (2012). *Grécko-slovenský slovník. Od Homéra po kresťanských autorov*. Lingea.

Pelikan, J. (1985). *Reformation of Church and Dogma*, vol. 4. (1300-1700), University of Chicago Press.

Pesch, O. H. (1968). *Thomas von Aquin. Grenzen und Größe mittelalterlicher Theologie*. Grünewald Verlag.

Ricoeur, P. (1960). Le "péché original": étude de signification. In *Eglise et Théologie*. Paris (pp. 11-30).

Ricoeur, P. (1971). *Die Felhbarkeit des Menschen. Phänomenologie der Schuld I*. Karl Alber Verlag.

Riceour, P. (1971). *Symbolik des Bösen. Phänomenologie der Schuld II*. Karl Alber Verlag.

Ricoeur, P. (1974). *Hermeneutik und Psychoanalyse. Der Konflikt der Interpretationen II*. Kösel Verlag.

Scharfenberg, J. (1968). *Sigmund Freud und seine Religionskritik als Herausforderung für den christlichen Glauben*. Vandenhoeck&Ruprecht.

Schleiermacher, F. (1999). *Der Christliche Glaube nach den Grundsätzen der Evangelischen Kirche im Zusammenhange dargestellt (1830/31)*. In Martin Redeker (ed.). De Gruyter.

Schwarz, R. (1968). *Vorgeschichte der reformatorischen Busstheologie*. (AKG 41). De Gruyter.

Sitzler-Osing, D. (1999). Schuld. In H. Balz, (ed.). *Theologische Realenzyklopädie* (TRE) XXX. De Gruyter (pp. 572-577).

Tillich, P. (1967). *Systematic Theology*. The University of Chicago Press.

Zálešák, T. (2005). *Diablova práca. Úvahy o totalitarizme*. Kalligram.

(In)justice
On the Indeterminacy
of the Concept of (In)justice

Olexij M. Meteňkanyč

> *Those who reproach injustice do so because they are afraid not of doing it but of suffering it. So, Socrates, injustice, if it is on a large enough scale, is stronger, freer, and more masterly than justice.*
>
> Thrasymachus in Plato, *Republic* 1.344c.

Introduction and (minor) historical context

It is not surprising that we begin our study of the concept of (in)justice with a quotation from Plato's *Republic,* a work that is still often referred to today when examining the simple-sounding question, *"What is justice?"* (Plato, *Republic,* 1.331b-c). Whole generations of readers could also become familiar with one of the greatest recorded debates about the nature of justice (specifically from Plato, *Republic,* 1.337b): the sophist Thrasymachus argued eristically about injustice, while Socrates tried to refute his arguments one by one. The well-known sophist points out that power and wealth are easily acquired by unjust actions. The chosen few, the smart and courageous, should not toil and strive in vain for a virtuous life when they can prosper through strength and subterfuge. Law and justice are mere tools "created" by the mediocre crowd, the weak and meek, who, at the hands of the powerful, merit not justice but disdain (Plato, *Gorgias,* 483b-d, 488). Many of us disagree with such a claim (following Socrates). We assume that justice is something better than injustice and that acting unjustly is actually the worst thing to do (Plato, *Gorgias,* 469b-c).

Many of us grow up with some version of this moral lesson. But interestingly, in adulthood, the effort to distinguish between justice and injustice (as concepts) is not given a significant amount of attention. Our mediatized political and ethical debates rarely address what exactly "is" justice and injustice. Rather, they tend to focus on specific manifestations and questions: Can war be seen as just? Is the killing of a human being an act of injustice in every circumstance? Is it just to prohibit abortion? Is it fair to open marriage and child-rearing to same-sex partners? We often take a pragmatic stance, and it seems that these issues can be decided without having to examine the concepts of justice and injustice in a broader sense. Perhaps we also believe that if we address specific problems, one by one, we will gradually achieve justice throughout society and eliminate injustice as something negative that burdens us as a society. While this may sound utopian, it underscores a fundamental point – the problem of (in)justice is omnipresent.

It is Plato´s *Republic* that is considered to be the first programmatic justice theory (Heinze, 2013, 5). Of course, many have followed up on this theme and made their mark on the history of thought by exploring the phenomena of justice and injustice. Two millennia of philosophy have constantly delivered theories aiming to exhaust the concept of (in)justice, to pin down its essence or core. From Plato´s disciple Aristotle, through thinkers such as Thomas Aquinas, John Locke, Jean-Jacques Rousseau, Immanuel Kant, G. W. F. Hegel, John Stuart Mill, and Karl Marx, to prominent 20th- and 21st-century thinkers such as John Rawls, Robert Nozick, Amartya Sen, Michael Walzer, Martha Nussbaum, Nancy Fraser, Axel Honneth, or Jürgen Habermas, to name a few. And yet, (in)justice is one of the key themes of human thought. It seems that we still lack a comprehensive and universally accepted definition of it. Indeed, some point out that the concepts of justice and injustice are paradoxical. On the one hand, they are everyday words, widespread throughout the world and used by everyone, intuitively understood by all of us, and even, if necessary, many of us can relate to them, and add attributes, aspects, and dimensions to them. On the other hand, however, humanity has struggled with the difficult task of clearly delineating and defining both concepts since their inception. Simultaneously, the paradoxicality is also linked to the fact that the notion of (in)justice is often not only a question of rationality but also a problem of emotionality and subjectivism (what is (in)just for me may not be for another), which has been aptly expressed by Ota Weinberger *"the pursuit of justice is a task of seeking, a task for the mind and the heart"* (Weinberger, 2010, 364).

It is remarkable that the complexity and difficulty of understanding the phenomenon of (in)justice (especially in legal discourse) has been pointed out for a long time. In the past, we have demonstrated the above by analyzing one of the most cited and accepted definitions of justice that can be found, namely in *Institutes of Justinian*, a codification of Roman Law from the 6th century AD (Meteňkanyč, 2023, 142–143). In *Institutes*, the justice is defined as *"the constant and perpetual will to render to each his due"*. It highlights important aspects of justice (justice and individual claims; justice and charity; justice and enforceable obligation; justice and impartiality; justice and agency, for more see Miller, 2021) and even on the basis of this short definition one can understand the complexity and considerable vagueness of justice, since there are many issues and uncertainties associated with the definition (for more see Meteňkanyč, 2023, 142 et seq.).

It is important to note that we will address both the concepts of justice and injustice, as we consider them to be closely intertwined, and examining one without the other could lead to a misleading view. Therefore, the subject matter of this study is an analysis of the reasons why the notions of justice and injustice are one of the vaguest notions, not only in the study of social and legal philosophy. One of the possible reasons that (in)justice is problematic and difficult to grasp is its potential multidimensionality. (In)justice is "saturated" from many areas and dimensions, and therefore it is often very difficult to wholly gather them under a single umbrella notion (as already hinted in the definition of justice in *Institutes*). We will attempt to focus on several reasons for the ambiguity of the concept of (in)justice and the terms we use to denote it, as well as the various ways that we can explore the concept of (in)justice. Initially, we will focus on the etymological aspects of the concept of (in)justice, noting that in some languages, the terms used to refer to (in)justice highlight different aspects than those highlighted by other languages (yet simultaneously it is possible to see certain overlaps, which we will point out). Subsequently, we will present another approach to the clarification and definition of terms used to label concepts through an analysis of their contents. There are two methods used to obtain meanings: the direct *a priori* definition of concepts and the indirect argument. We will attempt to define the terms "justice" and "injustice" by analyzing their synonyms (taken from dictionaries and common users – the direct approach) and their opposites (the indirect approach). Through this conceptual analysis of the synonyms of the terms "injustice" and "justice", we will try to outline the borders and plasticity of the semantic space of the mentioned terms and suggest their various semantic levels. Also, we believe that the meaning of terms cannot only be directly revealed but also indirectly – by illustrating the meaning of its opposites. Finally, in the last part of the study, we will attempt, from the perspective of selected disciplines (moral psychology and law), to reflect on the question of why the concept of (in)justice (or what it signifies) is important to us despite not being entirely clear or well definable.

The Concept of (In)justice and Its Etymological Aspects

If we look at the words used to designate "injustice" in various languages, we will see that the most basic words used to denote this concept are often derived from wholly different terms or etymological roots.

Looking at the English language, the term "injustice" has its roots in Latin and Old French, with a noticeable influence from classical Greek. The Latin word *"iniustitia"* serves as the direct precursor to *"injustice"*. It is a compound word consisting of "in-" (meaning "not" or "opposite of") and *"iustitia"* (in a meaning of "justice" or "righteousness", see Klein, 1966, 797). In Latin, *"iustitia"* is derived from *"ius"* (meaning "right", "that which is sanctioned or ordained, law" or "that which is just", or "that which is binding"; see Oxford Latin Dictionary, 1968, 984–985; Olivetti, 2024), and it refers to the quality of adherence to what is morally or legally right. Following this, the adjective "just" (in English) also refers to "morally upright, righteous in the eyes of God"; also "equitable, fair, impartial in one's dealings"; as well as "fitting, proper, conforming to standards or rules"; and "justifiable, reasonable"; from Old French *juste* "just, righteous; sincere" (12c.) and directly from Latin *iustus* "upright, righteous, equitable; in accordance with law, lawful; true, proper; perfect, complete" (Harper, 2024). Like many other words, the word "injustice" entered the English language via Old French. According to Online Etymology Dictionary (Etymonline. com), it came from the "injustice" in the late 14th century (Harper,

2024) and we can see that "injustice" in Old French retained its Latin roots, conveying the idea of *the absence or violation of justice* (so it denotes actions, behaviors, or situations that deviate from principles of fairness, equity, or moral rightness, leading to harm, inequality, or wrongdoing).[13]

Since we see that the base of the word "(in)justice" is derived from *"ius"*, it is appropriate to examine it in more detail. In his study of the etymological roots of words of "justice" and "judge", Jason Boatright (2018, 730–735) distinguishes four competing etymologies of the origin of *"ius"*, namely: Ad 1) *ius* as "command, fear, and violence". *"Ius"* posits that it came from the Latin word *"jussi"*, meaning "that which is ordained by laws human or divine"; *"jussi"* is a form of the Latin verb *"jubeo"*, meaning "I command" but etymologically two other related meanings are pointed out, namely "to frighten, and so frighten with menaces, menace, then to command in a menacing manner" and "battle, fight" (for more see Valpy, 1828, 212; de Vaan, 2008, 312).

Ad 2) *ius* as "need" and, perhaps, "request, distribution, and receipt". This explanation for the origin of *"ius"* is that it originated directly from the classical Greek adjective δεος (deos), meaning "right". However, the meaning itself is more likely to be interpreted as something "that is binding or necessary" (Valpy, 1828, 213; 1860, 35), and not in meaning of "just, or proper, or legal". Or as Boatright (2018, 732) simplistically puts it: "δεος or *"right"*, *is about what someone must do, rather than what someone may or should do"*. Also it is worth mentioning that the verb "δεω" (deo) can mean "to bind"; "to want, need, beg, [or] ask", or "to divide" (Valpy, 1860, 37).

Ad 3) *ius* as a "binding, a yoke". It is similar in meaning to the previous explanation (ii.), i.e., an idea of "joining" or "binding", but the third etymology contends *ius* is descended from the Sanskrit verb *yu*, meaning *"to join"* (Skeat, 1888, 309 and 725) (and not from

---

13 The most well-known English dictionaries see "injustice" in the same way: *Merriam-Webster Dictionary* (2024) explains "injustice" as an absence of justice (violation of right or of the rights of another) or an unjust act; *Cambridge English Dictionary* (2024) characterizes this term as a situation in which there is no fairness and justice or as a condition of being unfair and lacking justice, or an action that is unfair; and *Oxford Learner's Dictionaries* (2024) describes "injustice" as a fact of a situation being unfair and of people not being treated equally – an unfair act or an example of unfair treatment.

the Greek δεω). Verb *"yu"*, along with the Greek word "συω" (syo), meaning "to sew", are the root of the Old English *"yeoc"*, which is the modern English *"yoke"*. In this meaning, it is possible to interpret *ius* as an idea that we are bound or joined to the law, and therefore obligated by it (Halsey, 1889, 69-70).

Ad 4) finally, fourth etymology explains that *ius* came from the Proto Indo-European noun *"h2oiu"* or *"h2i-eu-s"* meaning "vital force, eternity" (de Vaan, 2008, 316-317), with connection to the Sanskrit nouns *"yoh"*, meaning "health", *"yos"* meaning *"of life"*, and *"ayus"* meaning "life span, life". Nouns h2oiu or h2i-eu-s are roots of the Greek word "ου", meaning "not", and Boatright (2018, 733) points out that "ου" developed from the concept of the "negation of energy", and a "limitation on eternity"; this view is supported by the fact that mentioned Sanskrit nouns *yoh, yos,* and *ayus* denote a temporary manifestation of energy and existence before its inevitable decay and annihilation (de Vaan, 2008, 316-317) and, therefore, they refer to something that is necessarily finite.

In summary, if we were to look for a common denominator of the etymologies described above, it would probably be about fact that the word *"ius"* descended from words *relating to restriction*. The command (and the associated meanings of fear and violence in the event of non-compliance with the command) indicates Subject A´s coercive influence on Subject B to do something that Subject B would not otherwise do. Similarly, if *"ius"* came from words denoting the distribution of rights and needs, it would be a matter of which subjects get them and which don´t. Likewise, if *"ius"* refers to words signifying obligation(s), it would be about restriction of freedom. Lastly, if *"ius"* were related to life or health, it would be in the sense that life and health has many limitations (including the moment of finitude). So, *"ius"* is tied up with the possibility of limitation, of placing certain boundaries, and whoever crosses them will be in contradiction with it will be *unjust*.

If we were to examine other languages that are based on Latin terminology (the Romance languages: Italian, Spanish, etc.), we would see similar etymological aspects of the concept of (in)justice. The etymological roots and original meaning of this term that comes from the Latin *"iustitia"* (Italian "giustizia", Spanish "justicia", Romanian "justiție" etc.) and have a similar semantic meaning as we have described above.

Simultaneously, when etymologically examining the term "(in)justice", it is worth mentioning that while the direct origin of "injustice" is Latin, the concept of (in)justice has deep roots in classical Greek philosophy. The ancient Greek word ἀδικία (adikia) is a compound word formed from the prefix ἀ- (a-), which signifies negation or absence, and the noun δίκη (dikē), usually meaning "justice" or "right". Therefore, ἀδικία (adikia) literally means "lack of justice" or "absence of righteousness", and word ἀδικέω (adikeo) can be translated as "to be unjust", "perpetrate injustice", "be wrong", or "violate the rules" (Montanari, 2015, 31-32). The noun δίκη (dikē) carries various meanings related to justice, judgment, and what is right or lawful. It can refer not only to legal judgments, court, decisions, legal actions, sentence, and penalty but also to a rule, custom, or a manner (Montanari, 2015, 530). Also, from noun δίκη different derivatives and compounds are formed in ancient Greek. For example, δικαίωμα (dikaiōma) refers to an act of justice, reparation (of wrong) or judgement; δικαίωσις (dikaiōsis) refers to the act of justification or vindication; or δικαιωτής (dikaiōtis) refers to a judge (Montanari, 2015, 530). These words share the root δικ- (dik-), which underlines their connection to concepts of justice and righteousness.

Bohuš Tomsa (2007, 64-68) in examining the word δίκη notes several meanings, namely (i) internal compulsion, custom, habit; (ii) necessity to which one is subject against one´s will; and (iii) righteousness. However, Tomsa points out that in its original meaning the word δίκη signified *a regularly recurring phenomenon*. And every such phenomenon attracts man´s attention because of its regularity, and tempts him to suppose that some intelligent coercive power, some purposeful will, is behind it. The ancient Greek paused at regularly reoccurring phenomena and was led to believe in the existence of a kind of premeditation or planfulness. And this premeditation and planfulness he saw in the whole of nature therefore seemed to him to be the only whole, behind which there was that intelligent higher power, causing by its intervention the remarkable order of all events – and this intelligent power he then called by the name δίκη (Tomsa, 2007, 65). Thus δίκη also had a cosmic meaning here, as the goddess of the world order, *indicating/pointing* in what direction not only man but all of nature should go. Her will was a law, demanding always for a certain case a certain way of behavior, i.e., a *regularity*, to which man had to submit (even against his will). Hence the word δίκαιος (dikaiōs) adjectivally meant "such as it ought to be", identical with that required by the higher natural order, hence δίκη also means that which is "appropriate to the natural course of things" (Tomsa, 2007, 66).

Martin Heidegger has his own unique view of the translation of δίκη. In *Introduction to Metaphysics* (1935), Heidegger offers *"fit/fittingness"* (*Fug*) as a translation for δίκη (Heidegger, 2000, 171), the term usually translated into German as *Gerechtigkeit* (*justice*).[14] Heidegger claims that when one translates δίκη as "justice" – and understands justice in a juridical-moral sense – then the word loses its fundamental metaphysical content (Heidegger, 2000, 171). Similarly, he is critical of the understanding of δίκη as a "norm", "right", or "law" (in the objective sense), since these are terms that reflect (only) legal or judicial understanding, but that fail to think the "overwhelming" dimension of being as what is uncanny and resistant to human control. Instead, Heidegger will think δίκη as belonging together with two other fundamental Greek terms: φύσις (physis) and λόγος (logos), thought in Heraclitus' sense (cf. Heidegger, 2000, 131 et seq.). As Heidegger claims: *"being, physis, is, as sway, originary gatheredness: logos. Being is fittingness that enjoins: dikē."* (Heidegger, 2000, 171). Heidegger goes on to say that this notion of being as δίκη (*Fug*) needs to be grasped in terms of its *"reciprocal relation"* to τέχνη (technē),[15] one where they are joined in the opposition between *"the excessive violence of being"* (*die Übergewalt des Seins*) and the human being's capacity for *"violence-doing"* (*die Gewalt-tätigkeit des Daseins;* cited as in Bambach, 2021, 441). In this violent confrontation that brings into play the counter-turning relation of δίκη and τέχνη, Heidegger finds a way

---

14 Heidegger understands fittingness first in the sense of joint and structure; then as arrangement, as the direction that the overwhelming gives to its sway; finally, as the enjoining structure, which compels fitting-in and compliance (Heidegger, 2000, 171).

15 In a meaning of "knowing". Τέχνη means neither art nor skill, and it means nothing like technology in the modern sense. According to Heidegger "knowing"/τέχνη here also does not mean the result of more observations about something present at hand that was formerly unfamiliar. Such items of information are always just accessory, even if they are indispensable to knowing. Knowing, in the genuine sense of τέχνη, means initially and constantly looking out beyond what, in each case, is directly present at hand (Heidegger, 2000, 169).

to express "the enjoining structure" (*das fügende Gefüge*) of being as φύσις that comes to language in the Heraclitean λόγος of cosmic order (Bambach, 2021, 441).

At the same time, according to Heidegger, it is necessary to distinguish between δίκη and *iustitia*. He emphasizes that *iustitia* has a wholly other essential ground than does δίκη. By translating δίκη as "justice" (in Latin *iustitia*) and placing it within the frame of a juridical-moral interpretation, Western thought completed a process begun by the Romans who translated δίκη as *iustitia* without experiencing the original meaning of Greek δίκη as a "showing" (δείκνῡμῐ/deiknymi), a "pointing toward" (δεῖξις/deixis) of the "pattern" or "sketch" (δεῖγμα/deigma) that being "brings to light" and "shows forth" (Bambach, 2021, 441). This etymological cluster of terms all belongs within the "phenomenological mode" of *indicating* and *pointing*, whereas the Latin translation of δίκη as *iustitia* has its roots in *ius* (mostly in a meaning of "law" and "right", "that which is sanctioned or ordained", "that which is just", or "that which is binding", as we mentioned above). Therefore, Heidegger was interested in justice understood as a particular style of the unfolding of *being* – namely, "*an order of being in an originary sense that is not preset or that overrides all entities in advance of what appears, but that emerges in and through the dynamic fit of oppositional tension between con-junction and dis-junction occurring in the singular joint of appearance*" (Bambach, 2021, 440). Within such an order of δίκη, "justice" is neither a legal nor moral arrangement or ordinance, but instead the fitting adjustment of each being to the fit of the play between δίκη (Fug/jointure) and ἀδικία (adikia/Un-Fug/disjointure). Hence, Heidegger will risk translating δίκη as *Fug*, in the sense of "what is fitting" that which, when it is joined together (*gefügt*), "fits" (Bambach, 2012, 243).[16]

In summary while the term "(in)justice" itself may have direct Latin origins, its conceptual exploration and development owe much to the foundational ideas of classical Greek philosophy and we should not overlook that there is a curious relationship between *(in)iustitia* and δίκη/ἀδικία that is worthy of further research.

---

16 Unfortunately, at this point we do not have the opportunity to address this issue in more detail; for more, we recommend to see Bambach (2012, 2021), Weston (2012), and Lemm (2013).

In some Slavic languages, we perceive certain similarities, but also differences in the etymological inquiry of "injustice". We can see that injustice (Russian "несправедливость", Polish "niesprawiedliwość", Slovak "nespravodlivosť", Croatian "nepravda", Serbian "неправда" etc.) is significantly interlinked to the term of "truth" (Russian and Serbian, "правда", Slovakian and Croatian "pravda", Polish "prawda"). Injustice, also in Slavic languages, is a compound word that contains the denotation of "justice" (e.g., Russian "справедливость", Polish "sprawiedliwość", Slovak "spravodlivosť", Croatian "Pravda"), and the prefix "не-" (ne-) is added. This prefix serves as a negation, similar to the English prefix "un-" or "in-". It denotes the reversal or absence of the quality expressed by the root word, in this case, justice.

Often the word "injustice" is not even explicitly mentioned in etymological dictionaries (see, for instance, Rejzek, 2001; Králik, 2015), and it is necessary to look at the word "justice", which is often associated with two meanings, namely *"truth"* ("pravda") and *"right"* ("pravý" as an adjective) (Ondruš, 2004, 13–14). We´ll start with the later one.

The etymological origin of the term "justice" (but also law) is also associated with the *"right side"*. The base of the word in Slavic languages is intertwined with the word "right" (e.g., *pravý - spravodlivý*) (Derksen, 2008, 418). The Proto-Slavic **prav* is probably from the Indo-European **prō-ųo-*, where **prō* is etymologically identical with the prefix *pra-, pro-*, the original meaning being apparently "in front/forwardly going", "facing forward", i.e. "direct", as opposed to "krivý" ("crooked/twisted"), whence the moral sense then came to use "správny, spravodlivý" ("right, just"), i.e., one who acts directly, without subterfuge, etc., or to be "the opposite of left", according to the fact that most people use their right hand for their main activities, hence this side is "správna" ("right"). This is also why injustice is most often associated with "wrongdoing" ("krivda"), i.e., one who has not acted in the "right" way has strayed from what should have been done, and has committed a misconduct, an offence (Králik, 2015, 466).

Similarly, in the development of Romance terminology, it can be seen that the original meaning of the word "rectus" (and the term "directus" derived from it) was *"straight, direct"* (in the physical sense of equality), the basis of this word being derived from the

Latin *"regere",* meaning "to lead", "to govern", or "to rule" (Špaňár and Hrabovský, 2012, 514). Only gradually, over time, did the meaning of the word shift secondarily to the moral-legal level of meaning "right, moral and good". In classical Latin, the term "rectus" denoted both the physical meaning of equality and directness, but also the moral-legal meaning of rightness, while later (in Vulgar Latin) the original meaning of physical equality is subsequently dropped and only the meaning of moral-legal rightness or morality remains (Špaňár and Hrabovský, 2012, 508). Out of this Latin cluster of terms with close etymological roots, we also find *rego*: "to rule" or "govern"; *regula*: in a meaning of "to set a pattern, rule, for example"; *regio*: "a boundary line" or "region"; as well as *reor*: in a meaning of "to reckon" or "think"; and of course *ratio*: "reason" (Bambach, 2012, 238). In Germanic languages we can observe a similar development, when the Germanic term "recht" had its original meaning in the form of physical equality, i.e., in the sense of "straight, direct". It was only by later developments in Old High German that it acquired, in addition to its original meaning of physical straightness, a moral-legal meaning in the form of "right, just, moral, impeccable" (Gábriš and Jáger, 2016, 102).

"Pravda" (truth) is in turn a derivative of **praviti* in the sense of "to make straight, direct". The original meaning of this word was perhaps a (proper) management, administration. Hence the older conception of "pravda" as "justice", "law", and further as the "administration of justice" (also in the form of a court of law). There is a known saying: "už je na pravde Božej" ("he/she is already in the truth of God", we can literally say that "už je na Božom súde = už stojí pred Božím súdom, už je mŕtvy" ("he/she is already at the court of God = he/she is already standing before God´s court, he/she is already dead") and the decision of God is coming. Just is that which "is with the truth" (Rejzek, 2001, 595). Hence the word *"rule"* – from **praviti*: "to make right, i.e. straight"; originally in relation to instruments (older "an instrument for measuring/keeping a straight course", e.g. this is true of a protractor, a spirit level, a rudder). "Správať sa" ("to behave") then, similarly, was originally based on the idea of being governed (by rules, conventions). This is followed by the word "právo" ("law"), which literally means "to pravé" ("the right thing"), in the sense of "direct, straight", "acting without subterfuge, according to justice", and has been used in this sense since about the 15th century (Králik, 2015, 466). Ján Doruľa also points out that the term "pravda" ("truth") was used in documents from the period of the Kingdom of Hungary primarily in the sense of the contemporary Slovak "justice", "legal order", or "court". He supports this conclusion not only with examples from preserved folklore but also with citations of specific historical documents (Doruľa, 1966, 307; 1972).

We should also add that the theory where the meaning of the terms "spravodlivosť" ("justice"), "pravda" ("truth"), and "právo" ("right") is to be derived from the original term denoting physical equality or directness can also be demonstrated in the development of the related paired words. The opposite of the term denoting physical equality *pravъ* was not only the term *levъ* ("left") but also the term *krivъ* ("crooked, curved"). And it is known that with the gradual development of the term *pravъ* changed into the derivative "pravda", also the term *krivъ* changed by the same development into the term "krivda" ("wrongdoing", "guilt"). Consequently, it is not surprising that the meaning of justice, correctness, or, on the contrary, the meaning of injustice, incorrectness, has also been acquired (Gábriš and Jáger, 2016, 103–104).

To add, the word *pravъ* has acquired a number of derivatives in Slavic languages over time; let us mention a few: *praviti:* "to govern", "to administer", later also "to speak" ("hovoriť"), *pravota* ("righteousness", "rightness"); *pravilьnъ* ("correct"), *pravitelь* ("leader"), *pravljenije* ("rule of conduct", "justice"), *ispraviti* ("to make straight", "to correct", "to direct"), *ispravitelь* ("corrector", "guide"), but also for us the key derivative, namely the term "*pravъda*", which in Old Slavonic had the meaning of "rule", "law", or even today's meaning of "truth", but perhaps the most common was the meaning of "justice".[17] According to Ondruš, the Old Slavonic *pravьda* corresponded in meaning to the Greek δίκαιον (dikaion), ἀλήθεια (aletheia) and the Latin *iustitia* and *veritas* (Ondruš, 2004, 19).

Naturally, much more could be written on the etymology of the concept of (in)justice. We could also look at other words that

---

17 For a comparison of translations of selected documents of the Great Moravian period that contain the term pravьda see more in Gábriš and Jáger (2016, 105–108).

denoted justice in other ancient cultures. From Sumerian *"me"* to Accadian *"kittu"*, Ancient Egyptian *"maat"*, or Ancient Indian *"r(i) ta, dharma"*, it is acknowledged that all the above-mentioned roots and their derivatives reflect the primeval adjustment of the human being to communication and harmony (Krašovec, 2015, 314). However, it is apparent that the concept of (in)justice has different etymological roots of individual words, which, although they have selected common aspects, at the same time, also have several differences, which leads to the conclusion that the concept in question is multidimensional and meaningfully polysemic. In some languages, the terms used to refer to (in)justice highlight different aspects than those highlighted by other languages. Ordinary users of languages in their own contexts of meaning may not experience this difference/ambiguity as a problem in everyday communication, but it would be more difficult if we were to try to establish the international limits of the meaning of the concept of (in)justice in an exact way. This may be the reason that we do not fully understand each other when discussing concepts of (in)justice, as we are not always referring to the same thing. It is not surprising to state that our concepts often aim to express different meanings. However, the foregoing implies that it is not only necessary to stick to etymological or linguistic inquiry, but it is advisable to look for and map the semantic meanings that are denoted by the various "(un)just" concepts and deduce what a particular language user has in mind. To put it differently, we also want to engage in a semantic analysis of the concept of (in)justice.

Semantics of the Concept of (In)justice

How is it actually possible to explore the semantic levels of the concept of (in)justice, when it is obvious even to an ordinary language user that this concept encompasses many, often different, levels and dimensions? In this respect, we want to build on the progress of several recent studies (Démuth and Démuthová, 2023a, 30–34; Démuth, Démuthová and Keceli, 2023, 42–48; Kišoňová, 2023, 94–97; Batka, 2023, 103–109; Krašovec, 2015) that address diverse conceptions of emotions using semantic analysis. By it, we mean the analysis of the meaning of concepts in natural language by examining their relationships (semantic and extensional similarities and differences) to related (similar and opposite) concepts in the given language. Such analysis assumes the exploration of intersections, as well as the semantic differentiation of the examined concepts, their disambiguation, and the examination of their mutual relationships (Démuth and Démuthová, 2023a, 32). In this regard, it is possible to carry out an analysis of concepts that can be partially subsumed under the notion of (in)justice in a particular language, here it is appropriate to use a conceptual analysis of synonymous and antonymous terms.

Starting with injustice, whereby if we review the most famous English dictionaries (Thesaurus, 2024; Cambridge Dictionary, 2024; Oxford Dictionary, 2024; Collins Dictionary, 2024), some of the most common synonyms for injustice include: unfairness; unjustness; imbalance; inequity; discrimination; partiality; abuse; breach; bias; favoritism; bigotry; prejudice; oppression; one-sidedness; violation; exploitation; foulness; wrong; wrongdoing; negligence; injury; crime; malpractice; error; damage; offense; persecution; encroachment; unfairness; insult; sin; evil; grievance; abuse; misdeed, foul play; outrage.

Similarly, the *Dictionary of Slovak Synonyms* (2004) lists words such as krivda (wrongdoing, grievance), bezprávie (lawlessness); neprávosť (wrong); príkorie (iniquity, wrongdoing); ústrk (wrong in a meaning of pushback, pushing away); zlo (evil); protivenstvo (adversity); neprávo (unlaw).

At the same time, the most frequent antonyms for the word "injustice" are justice; equity; fairness; fair play; impartiality; lawfulness; rectitude; right; righteousness; equality; cheer; delight; good deed; happiness; joy; kindness; obedience; respect; equitableness; tolerance (Thesaurus, 2024; Cambridge Dictionary, 2024; Oxford Dictionary, 2024).

It is clearly mentioned that synonyms capture different aspects of injustice, such as unfair treatment, unequal distribution of resources, discrimination based on various factors like race or gender, and the abuse of power or authority. They highlight situations where fairness is lacking, rights are violated, and individuals or groups are subjected to unfairness or disadvantage. Depending on the context, some of these synonyms may be more appropriate than others in describing specific instances or forms of injustice. For instance, injury, wrong, and grievance are comparable when they denote an act that inflicts undeserved damage, loss, or hardship on a person. Injury applies to an injustice to a person for which the law allows an action to recover compensation or specific property (or both); wrong is, in law, a more general term than injury for it applies not only to all injuries as defined above (as a private wrongs) but also to all misdemeanors or crimes which affect the community (*public wrongs*) and which are punishable according to the law. Grievance applies to a circumstance or condition that, in the opinion of those affected, constitutes a wrong or that gives one just grounds for complaint (Webster´s New Dictionary of Synonyms, 1973, 447).

We believe that the concept of injustice encompasses the following conceptual aspects:

Ad 1/ words such as unfairness, imbalance, discrimination, partiality, abuse, bias, and favoritism indicate that the essence of injustice is the violation of a just principle or equality. It may occur in different contexts, such as legal systems, social interactions, or the distribution of resources, but there will be some apparent imbalance in the status quo. It is a disruption of the harmony that was initially established. In simple terms, we can say that it is "a state of being unfair or unjust".

Ad 2/ injustice, of course, can also be tied not only to the state but also to the act itself. An unjust act emphasizes a moment of undesirability in society, since it is a disregard for the moral principle of acting equally toward all, or a disregard for the rights of others, which is (often) also linked to the consequence that some harm to others will occur. Often, therefore, the above is associated with words of the type "wrong, crime, offense, insult, sin, grievance, or misdeed".

Ad 3/ simultaneously, an important aspect of injustice relates to the moment of impairment of impartiality (often in litigation), or we can describe it as a failure to observe the principles of impartial evaluation. The existence of rules of conduct often presupposes that those who are supposed to supervise compliance with the rules will do so independently, impartially, objectively, in accordance with agreed procedural rules, ensuring that adequate punishment is subsequently meted out if a violation of a right, equality, or other just principle is indeed established. However, this presupposes a process that is not unfair, discriminatory, biased, illegal, abusive, corrupt, preferring, and favoring one outcome, bigoted or/and subjective.

Ad 4/ injustice is very much about perception; it is about the subjective rumination of diverse experiences and incidents, where one person perceives something as unjust that another person may not necessarily even perceive as unjust. At the same time, he or she perceives the experience as an injustice on his or her part, which he or she points to in society to seek reparation for the perceived injustice. Therefore, it is possible to notice that some synonyms emphasize this aspect (unjustness, violation, outrage, one-sidedness, exploitation, persecution, etc.).

Ad 5/ to conclude, we should add that closely linked to injustice is the moment of the need to cope with it by means of some kind of response (most often the use of sanctioning mechanisms). Injustice should not go unnoticed and must be dealt with (ideally corrected, mitigated, or eliminated) when it occurs. Synonyms like oppression, wrong, persecution, violation, (to stop) abuse, (preventing) foul play indicate this aspect of injustice as well. However, we should stress that it may not always be a moment of punishment in response to injustice; sometimes there may be a more profound aspect of compensation.

For a systematic comparison, we will also note the synonymous and antonymous terms of the concept of justice. Some of the most common synonyms for justice include righteousness, goodness, probity, right, uprightness, fairness, fair play, fair-mindedness, rightness, justness, due process, equity, equitability, equitableness, honor, truth, honesty, integrity, virtue, legality, right, proper cause, legitimacy, lawfulness, the law, constitutionality, justification, due punishment, reparation, penalty, sentence, chastisement, correction, atonement, amends, redress, satisfaction, just deserts, compensation, payment, remuneration (Thesaurus, 2024; Cambridge Dictionary, 2024; Oxford Dictionary, 2024).

Similarly, the *Dictionary of Slovak Synonyms* (2004) lists words such as neutralita, neutrálnosť (neutrality); nestrannosť (impartiality, nonpartisanship); nezaujatosť (disinterestedness); objektivita (objectivity); súdnictvo/justícia (judiciary/justice).

At the same time, the most frequent antonyms for the word justice are dishonesty, favoritism, inequity, injustice, partiality, unfairness, unlawfulness, unreasonableness, bias, untruth, wrong, harm, crime, corruption, one-sidedness (Thesaurus, 2024; Cambridge Dictionary, 2024).

Similarly, for the concept of justice, we can observe the following conceptual signs, which, in our opinion, result from the analysis of the presented synonyms and antonyms of the term justice:

1/ justice is significantly related to how particular people are treated (already mentioned claim: *"to each his due"*); typically, issues of justice arise in circumstances in which people can advance claims (to their rights, freedoms, opportunities, resources, etc.) but they can be potentially conflicting, and if so, we appeal to justice to resolve such conflicts by determining what each person is properly entitled to have.

2/ certainly, an essential aspect of justice is the fact that it often involves the fair treatment of individuals or groups, ensuring that decisions, actions, or outcomes are unbiased and impartial. However, it should be borne in mind that the criterion of fairness is still problematic today. It does not always mean treating everyone exactly the same. Instead, it often involves recognizing and addressing differences in circumstances, needs, and contributions (consequently, diverse theories of justice are formed). While equality aims for sameness, equity strives for fairness by allocating resources or opportunities according to individual circumstances to achieve a more just outcome.

3/ a frequently emphasized condition for establishing justice in society (in the sense of fairness described above) is impartiality. Thus, the administration of justice presupposes impartial decision-making without favoritism, discrimination, or personal prejudice, and thus judgments and actions in society should be based on objective criteria and well-researched relevant facts, and not on subjective opinions or preferences, which entails a moment of arbitrariness. Justice should be the opposite of arbitrariness. It was also interesting for us to discover that the *Dictionary of Slovak Synonyms* strongly ties justice to the meaning of neutrality, impartiality, and objectivity, but it does not further list other synonyms that are commonly found in English dictionaries.

4/ it is clear from what has been said so far that justice is linked to the proper administration of law (including the subjective rights of the individual) and justice (words such as legality, lawfulness, justness, due process, right, legitimacy accentuate this aspect). It is a meaning that is related to "maintenance of what is just or right by the exercise of authority or power". Justice pertains to the fair and equitable resolution of disputes, often involving punishment for wrongdoing and protection of individual rights. Therefore, administration of justice demands strict attention and obedience, due to the establishment of order in society, where failure to respect the administration of justice thus set-up will be referred to as *obstruction of justice* (creating a literal obstacle that obstructs justice, usually an act from outside the system) or *miscarriage of justice* (in a meaning a failure of a court or judicial system to come to a just conclusion, and therefore it is more of a failure in the administration of justice within the system). This aspect can be aptly described in legal practice: if we have two identical or similar cases, the court´s treatment of them should be the same. It emphasizes two fundamental attributes of the application of the law, namely the predictability of the law and its relative permanence (and at the same time, it is a rough formulation of the principle of legal certainty). Not surprisingly, this aspect is also intertwined with the concept of the rule of law: it is not to be governed by the arbitrary will of individuals or groups but by the rule of rational impersonal (legal) rules (Mrva, 2018, 99).

5/ however, the administration of justice itself presupposes certain requirements that are imposed on it, most often:

(1) consistency, i.e. coherence in the application of agreed rules, norms, or procedures. The whole concept of the rule of law and the principle of legal certainty also operates on the idea that similar cases should be treated in the same way, thereby ensuring predictability and avoiding arbitrary or discriminatory results.

(2) consistency promotes a moment of transparency in decision-making processes, with the aforementioned emphasis on quality reasoning by decision-makers to make their decisions precise, to clearly and convincingly justify the reasons for the decision, and to be open to potential criticism from interested parties, and possibly from wider society as well.

(3) the need to ensure access to justice, i.e. to ensure that all members of society have equal access to legal remedies, legal protection, and the possibility of redress (particularly relevant when society suffers from significant economic disparities between social groups, or when systemic discrimination occurs).

6/ a significant aspect is being "amenable to justice". It is a condition or state of being susceptible to justice. This indicates justice is necessarily something that is applied to or impressed upon the recipient by someone or something else.

7/ with the aspect "being amenable to justice" other aspects of justice are also associated, and these can be formulated as "assignment of deserved reward or punishment" or "punishment of an offender or retribution deemed appropriate for a crime/wrong" (see also Oxford English Dictionary, 2024). With the administration of justice, it is necessary to associate the moment of reaction to the occurrence of its observance (deserved reward) and also its violation (appropriate punishment). From the very beginning of the use of the term "justice", this aspect has been associated with it. The first written record of *"justice"* in England dates from 1137 (Oxford English Dictionary, 2024, I.2.a.). A historical record in the Anglo-Saxon Chronicle attributed to "a Monk of Peterborough" (Manly, 1916, 1) describes the King of England arresting three nobles suspected of treason, but subsequently releasing and pardoning them after they had paid homage to him. When the king released them, the nobles tricked the king again and took advantage of the fact that he did not punish them. The chronicle describes the above as "Þa *the suikes undergæton ðat he milde man was and softe ... and na justise ne dide*, þa *diden hi alle wunder*", which (roughly) means, *"when the traitors perceived that he (*i.e., the king) *was a mild man and soft ... and enforced no justice, then they did all wonder"* (Manly, 1916, 1). Here, the word "justice" does clearly refer to the meaning of "punishment of an offender or retribution deemed appropriate for a crime/wrong", together with "exercise of authority or power in maintenance of right".[18]

---

18 The Chronicle goes on to explain that the King's failure to punish the traitors encouraged other nobles to defy him, which undermined royal authority for the rest of his reign. And according to Jason Boatright in this way, the first recorded use of the word *justice* in English retains the original, precise meaning of *ius* (and

8/ finally, we would add that at the same time, justice, from our point of view, includes an aspect of adequate balance, which brings the use we make of our rights, privileges, and our duties into harmony, and moderates and tempers the strictness of the law (Ramshorn, 1839, 275). The moderation itself is often done with reference to humanity or decency (Števček, 2018, 48–52).

Obviously, we could continue and write at length in the above-mentioned efforts to grasp justice.19 Nevertheless, we believe that on the basis of the above, it is also possible to glimpse the basic semantic aspects of the concepts of justice and injustice. However, it is worth pointing out that many do not want to see injustice as a mere "negation" of the concept of justice. At first glance, the concepts of justice and injustice in everyday practice seem indeed to pair off logically, reflecting both their shared etymology and the dictionary definitions. Particularly in law, we work extensively within the justice/injustice binary, and traditional legal approaches perpetuate conventionally dualistic assumptions about injustice as the negation of justice and justice as the negation of injustice. And this is largely sufficient for our (everyday) grasp of the phenomena of (in)justice. In many habitual contexts, it is sufficient to speak of justice and injustice as opposites, and this is sufficient for ethical or legal discussions. But that approach can be problematized, and a number of scholars have done so.

In this regard, we can mention the work of Eric Heinze, who in his book *The Concept of Injustice* presents a series of arguments that seek to problematize the relationship between the concepts of justice and injustice as a negation of each other. Traditionally (and also following the etymology of the notion of justice/injustice), injustice has been perceived binary as the negation of justice, and a characteristic feature of the theories of many well-known thinkers (from Plato and Aristotle, to Aquinas, Locke, Kant, Mill, to Marx

---

then justice): restrictive or corrective action, the absence of which promoted behavior that would have required more restriction or correction (Boatright, 2018, 738).

19 One can also mention the way justice is understood through contrasting concepts, typically conservative vs. ideal justice, corrective vs. distributive justice, procedural vs. substantive justice, legal vs. ethical justice, comparative vs. non-comparative justice, deontological vs. consequentialist justice, etc. See more on this in Klabouch (1995), Schmidtz (2016), Miller (2011), or Weinberger (2017).

and Rawls) is that they explain injustice by assuming that it is necessary to identify a certain (theoretical) model of justice, so that anything that contradicts or negates this model as a whole, or an essential component of it, or negates it as such, will by definition be considered to be injustice. But it is suggested that we overlook the scope and complexity of injustice, impoverishing our understanding, if we merely consider the traditional mode of etymology and theoretically understand injustice as the complete negation of something else (the theoretical definition of justice).

For instance, Heinze argues that injustice as not justice may suggest a conceptually prior notion of justice, but feelings of injustice originate often in visceral responses. They largely lack any sense of antecedent or distinctly formulated concepts of justice. Notwithstanding etymology, it is often injustice, not justice, that represents the primordial, gut experience (Heinze, 2013, 28). He even goes further and proposes that if the two terms must be linked by an etymological binary (which is often emphasized), then it would seem more appropriate to "reverse the etymology" and make "injustice" an experientially primary term and "justice" its more abstract, theoretical derivative (Heinze, 2013, 28). It may be pointed out that injustice does not only include everything that does not already fall into the category of "justice". And while it is possible to find relations of simple opposition (and mutual exclusion) between the concepts of justice and injustice, as suggested above, at the same time there can and do arise situations where these relations become more complex, especially when broader socio-political contexts that matter substantially are brought into the picture.

Simultaneously, from Heinze's perspective, it seems wrong to maintain any assumption that some clear and well-conceived theory of justice must first be provided that would allow us to perform a prior mental negation in order to understand where the negative aspects of injustice lie. On the contrary, it is rather our sense of injustice that stakes out the ontologically and conceptually prior moment, and from which we arguably proceed to theorize about justice (Heinze, 2013, 42). If we were to ask the question, "What is injustice?" the answer should not be "Injustice is not the opposite of justice", although it will come close. Rather, the conclusion should be: "Injustice is not solely the opposite of justice, even if it is merely and simply the opposite in certain conventional senses" (Heinze, 2013, 8).

Reasons To Use the Concept of (In)Justice[20]

Regardless of the specific levels or final dimensions of the concept of (in)justice, it seems certain that the concept of (in)justice represents a general concept. Justice and injustice are truly multidimensional and complex notions of human thinking. They are overarching concepts, enriched by several dimensions and terms which are interrelated but does not merge. We can see moral-juridical, phenomenological, ontological, or other diverse ethical conceptions of (in)justice that make it difficult to grasp. So why is (in)justice such an essential concept if we cannot precisely define it and fully understand it? We will offer two perspectives/justifications, where it is obvious that we do not know exactly what this phenomenon is in its essence, but this does not prevent us from making it a "pillar" of a given area of the functioning of our society.

The Concept of (In)Justice in Legal Thought

It is noteworthy that many legal theorists´ definitions of (in)justice emphasize the importance of grasping the problem through the prism of intuition and as something we cannot clearly define. Viktor Knapp, perhaps the most prominent theorist of law in the second half of the 20th century in Czechoslovakia, refers to the concept of justice as *"intuitively comprehensible, but defining it causes considerable difficulty"* (Knapp, 1995, 86). Ota Weinberger highlights the well-known paradox of the relationship between law and justice when he states that *"a legal life is unthinkable without discussions about justice. The pursuit of a specific conception of justice is evident in every legal system. (...) What is "truly" just, however, is still more or less contested. (...) I am thus of the opinion that no one knows or is able to prove what is just."* (Weinberger, 2017, 226–227).

---

[20] We have previously discussed selected ideas in this chapter elsewhere, see also Metenkanyč (2023) for a more comprehensive elaboration.

Even Hans Kelsen, a well-known representative of continental legal positivism, thinks of justice as an irrational ideal, which, on the one hand, is indispensable for human will and behavior but, on the other hand, is inaccessible to human cognition (Kelsen, 1933, 13). The irrational roots of justice for us were clearly expressed at the end of the 20th century by Jiří Klabouch when he stated, *"(...) the search for justice is not really about conflicts of ideas (...), but about the fluctuations of some very intense and deeply rooted emotions"* (Klabouch, 1995, 559). From our perspective, the contribution of Klabouch's theorem lies primarily in the distinction between the irrationality and the emotional force or significance (existential dimension) of justice attitudes and evaluations. These are important to human beings, and feelings of (in)justice are among the subjectively significant ones. At the same time, they do not emerge from the rationale, even though they are often later elaborated, articulated, organized, and eventually enforced by it.

Even today, literally after millennia of exploring the relationship between justice and law, many recent authors (cf. Bárány, 2011, 846; Kluknavská, 2021, 7) point to the fact that both legal thinking and legal practice do indeed work with justice, but with it as an undefined/indeterminate concept, despite the fact that legal scholarship usually precisely defines its concepts (especially in the Slovak region, where normativist and dogmatic legal thinking still plays a significant role). Bárány justifies the above with reference to two arguments in particular: (i) while legal thinking often uses the notion of justice, and it plays an important role in it, legal thinking respects that it is neither a legal nor a legal-philosophical notion. It leaves its definition primarily to social philosophy, from which legal theory draws when considering the concept of justice; (ii) justice is based on intuitions of what is (un)just, and in this sense "escapes" legal-theoretical knowledge (Bárány, 2011, 846).

However, this does not prevent us from postulating the requirement of justice in law, including at the level of not only its creation but also its implementation (with an emphasis on the application of the law), and at the same time the law reflects the needs and functions of justice, where it distinguishes its several forms and divisions (Weinberger, 2017, 229–233). And while it does not precisely define the concept of justice itself, despite this fact and the variety of approaches to justice, it is possible to infer a common understanding of justice (let´s call it a *"consciousness of justice"*), certain shared foundations that are implicitly (and intuitively) present in it, and legal thinking builds on these foundations (Weinberger, 2017, 229; Bárány, 2011, 847). Yet, let us not forget that it is characteristic of legal thought that it links law to a certain type of theories of justice, namely formal ones. In particular, this can be detected in the postulates of the "fair" application of the law, namely: (i) the principle of formal equality (i.e., that the law and its implementation are based on a general rule of law); (ii) the postulate of true fact-finding (what is established by law as a consequence of certain conditions can only be just if the requirement of true fact-finding is met, which is, however, a rather difficult requirement to meet in legal practice in certain cases); (iii) the postulate of implementation (rules are not only the basis for legal value judgments but also regulate conduct); (iv) the postulate of fair procedure (the justification for this postulate rests on the belief that by appropriately organizing the legal procedure, the probability of reaching a fair decision can be maximized, for more see Weinberger, 2017, 232).

It is also clear from our previous semantic analysis that justice is a relational concept, and this aspect is more evident in law. Fundamentally justice-oriented attitudes, evaluations, and intuitions are often transferable to solutions to the question of who is or should be (in)equal to whom in what. By injustice, then, we mean that there has been some kind of imbalance, a disruption of the "harmony" that was originally established. According to Bárány (2011, 853), justice is a relational concept in at least three meanings:
- primarily links what is judged to be (un)just, such as a legal norm, with the part of morality concerning the distribution of goods and burdens;
- the second meaning consists in connecting what is evaluated as (un)just with the irrationality, or rather the extra-rationality, of the just intuitions underlying morality, including its part concerning the distribution of goods and burdens; at the end of the chain of rational inference, there remains to be answered a question to which there is no longer a rational answer, although the answer to it is often taken for granted and trivial;
- the third meaning of the relationality of justice arises from the connection of the level of existential experiences with what is evaluated as (un)just, again, for example, the law.

In sum, although we do not really have a precise and universally accepted definition of (in)justice in legal thought today, and we work with the category in a rather intuitive way, the above does not mean that, thanks to the extensive debates on justice, we do not have at least an implicitly close understanding of the notion of (in)justice at our disposal in most cases. And the non-explicitness of the definition of justice is consequently not such a fundamental problem, since for many legal thinkers of different backgrounds and orientations in our Central European space, an important (if not crucial) component of justice is the irrational (extra-rational) basis of justice-oriented ideas, evaluations, and attitudes.

(In)Justice as an "Elicitor" of Moral Emotions

Since the late 20th century, we have seen a large body of work begin to be produced within neuroscience, social psychology, and cognitive studies that point to the importance of automatic and intuitive processes (to name a few, authors such as Haidt, Kahneman, Tversky, and others). Haidt, in his book *The Righteous Mind*, describes this shift as "new synthesis" and presents the following three principles: (1) Intuitions come first, strategic reasoning second; (2) There's more to morality than harm and fairness; (3) Morality binds and blinds (2012, chapters 2–4). Haidt explains these automatic and intuitive processes by using a now-famous metaphor: the mind is divided like a rider on an elephant, and the rider's job is to serve the elephant. The current view in psychology is that there are two basic and fundamentally different sorts of mental processes going on at all times in our minds: automatic processing (the elephant) and controlled processing (the rider).[21] Automatic cognition, symbolized by the great elephant, is sometimes referred to as "hot cognition". This is because it has the ability to nudge us into action; it is reactive and intuitive. Controlled cog-

---

21 "*Most of human cognition is like that of other animals. All brains are neural networks, and they solve problems largely by pattern matching. This sort of process happens rapidly and automatically. When you open your eyes, you recognize objects and faces. You don't have to do any conscious work; your visual system just solves ferociously difficult computational problems nearly instantaneously, and it presents its results to your conscious awareness.*" (Haidt, 2013, p. 869).

nition, on the other hand, is referred to as "cool cognition" since it is not connected to the behavioral centers of the brain. And in this respect, Haidt recommends us to imagine the human mind as a small and somewhat ineffectual rider perched on the back of a large, powerful, and rather smart elephant. *"The rider can try to steer the elephant, and if the elephant has no particular desire to go one way or the other, it may listen to the rider. But if it has its own desires, it's going to do what it wants to do"* (Haidt, 2013, 870).[22]

It is interesting to note, on the basis of the functioning of the human mind thus portrayed, that throughout the history of philosophy and thinking (and this includes the legal one), reason (i.e., the rider) has been appreciated. Within moral philosophy, in moral reasoning, there are many claims that the rider should always have complete control over the elephant, i.e., the controlled cognition has control over the automated one (e.g., see Kohlberg, 1973). To put it differently: rationalist approaches in moral psychology say that moral knowledge and moral judgment are reached primarily by a process of reasoning and reflection (Kohlberg, 1969; Piaget, 1932/1965). Intuition and moral emotions (such as sympathy, anger, guilt) may sometimes be inputs to the reasoning process, but they are not the direct causes of moral judgments. Reason and controlled cognition will eventually prevail.

However, Haidt (2013) suggests, based in part on a study of the writings of David Hume, that this is not the case. Reluctant to use similes like Hume when he described reason as a "slave of the passions" (Hume, 1739/2008), he interestingly enough chooses the comparison of reason as a press secretary. *"The press secretary*

---

[22] Kahneman and his colleagues describe these processes a little differently and refer to the above ways of thinking as System 1 and System 2 (see Kahneman, 2011, 19 et seq.; Kahneman and Klein, 2009, 515–526). S1 is "fast" thinking and produces *"effortlessly originating impressions and feelings that are the main sources of the explicit beliefs and deliberate choices of System 2"* and is mainly characterized by low mental energy consumption and is used in most of our everyday activities and tasks, in solving which we use familiar and used thought processes, and these processes are subconscious and fast (Kahneman, 2011, s. 21 et seq.). In turn, is our "slower" thinking. In contrast to S1 *"the highly diverse operations of System 2 have one feature in common: they require attention and are disrupted when attention is drawn away"* (Kahneman, 2011, 22). It is necessary to understand that S2 not only costs us a lot of time and requires full concentration (which distracts us from our other activities), but it also costs us a lot of mental strength.

of a president serves the president, but it's a partnership. Her job is not to figure out the truth, or to make policy; it is to justify whatever the president and his cabinet have decided to do" (Haidt, 2013, 871). The press secretary may have considerable influence on the running of the president and the "executive" and be a trusted advisor, but the president still runs everything. He or she will ultimately have to make the key decisions, but an important role of the press secretary is to develop and present arguments that portray the decisions in question to the public in the best light, in an effort to convince others of the justification for their implementation.

Subsequently, Haidt develops The Social Intuitionist Model, which is based on Hume´s model of intuitionism, but with newer terminology and with an overlap into society. The central claim of the model is that moral judgment is caused by quick moral intuitions and is followed (when needed) by slow, *ex post* facto moral reasoning (Haidt, 2001, 817–819). What is interesting is the social feature of this model. The social intuitionist model proposes that moral judgment should be studied as an interpersonal process. According to Haidt, moral reasoning is usually an *ex post facto* process used to influence the intuitions (and hence judgments) of other people (2001, 814). When reflecting on some negative phenomenon (e.g., incest, war), we usually immediately (intuitively) feel that it is something wrong.

However, when the societal need to justify this position is placed upon us (especially when the case becomes more complex and complicated), even the layperson must subsequently put himself or herself in the role of a judge, embrace the "case", and build an argument around his/her feelings. However, it is questionable with how much success, especially in interaction with others. And simultaneously, if he or she runs out of arguments, subsequently the familiar comes up: "I don't know, I can't explain it, I just know it's wrong." In a difficult debate, the above-mentioned often foreshadows defeat in argumentation; however, within the social intuitionist model, it becomes plausible to say it.

And after this minor introduction, we can proceed to the feeling of (in)justice and its understanding in contemporary moral psychology within the concept of moral emotions.

Justice experience does not only include cold cognition function of justice but also include hot emotion-laden responses to justice (Li, Hou, He, and Ma, 2022). We know that experiencing justice results in positive emotions such as joy, pride, pleasure, and so on (Weiss, Suckow, and Cropanzano, 1999). However, injustice has been often described as a kind of hot and burning experience, and even third parties respond strongly to injustice (O'Reilly, Aquino, and Skarlicki, 2016). The emotional experiences of (in)justice do not only affect attitude and behavior at individual level but also affect intergroup attitude and behavior at the group level. Experiencing justice or injustice, however, is not usually understood as a moral emotion. Moral emotions are defined as those emotions "that respond to moral violations or that motivate moral behaviour" (Haidt, 2003, p. 853). So, they are associated with social norms and values and the interests or welfare of persons or groups, beyond the concerns of the actors. That is, moral emotions function as signals of normative behavior (see Hareli, Moran-Amir, David, and Hess, 2013).

Nowadays, there are many classifications of moral emotions. Eisenberg (2000) at first proposed two kinds of moral emotions: self-conscious moral emotions (guilty, shame) and empathy. Lately, Haidt (2003) classified moral emotions into four kinds/families: those are self-conscious emotions (shame, embarrassment, and guilt), other-condemning emotions (contempt, anger, and disgust), other-suffering emotions (distress at another's distress, and sympathy), and other-praising emotions (gratitude, awe, and elevation). Gray and Wegner proposed a different approach to defining moral emotions. They both believe that "people divide the moral world along the two dimensions of valence (help/harm) and moral type (agent/patient). The intersection of these two dimensions gives four moral exemplars – heroes, villains, victims, and beneficiaries – each of which elicits unique emotions. For example, victims (harm/patient) elicit sympathy and sadness. Dividing moral emotions into these four quadrants provides predictions about which emotions reinforce, oppose, and complement each other" (Gray and Wegner, 2011). We are currently encountering also this division of emotions: positive self-conscious moral emotion (pride), negative self-conscious moral emotion (shame, guilt), positive other-focused moral emotion (elevation, grateful), negative other-focused moral emotion (anger, disgust, contempt, compassion; see more in Horberg, Oveis and Keltner, 2011; Rudolph and Tscharaktschiew, 2014). Rudolph, Schulz, and Tscharaktschiew (2013) conducted a comprehensive literature search to identify those emotions that have been labeled as moral emotions by scientists. It showed that during the past 100 years, about two dozen emotion terms have been labeled as moral emotions. These are, in alphabetical order: admiration, anger, awe, contempt, disgust, elevation, embarrassment, empathy, envy, gratitude, guilt, indignation, jealousy, pity, pride, rage, regret, remorse, resentment, respect (including self-respect), schadenfreude (joy in the misfortune of others), scorn, shame, and sympathy (compassion). But as we can see, neither justice nor injustice is mentioned here.

It is for this reason that perceived (in)justice is more often viewed as a triggering event (elicitor) for moral emotions. As we mentioned justice perception elicits positive moral emotions such as pride, pleasure, and so on, and injustice perception activates strong negative emotions such as anger, disgust, and contempt. Also, favorable unfair treatment triggers shame and guilt (Weiss, Suckow and Cropanzano, 1999; Rudolph and Tscharaktschiew, 2014; Tangney, Stuewig, and Mashek, 2007; Li et al., 2022). In the past, also Homans (1961) argued that people feel anger when they are underrewarded and guilt when they are overrewarded. Significant in experiencing (especially) injustice is the aspect of actor/observer, or we can say first- and third-person perspective criterion. A wide range of studies suggests that people evaluate and respond not only to the (in)justice they personally experience but also to the (in)justice experienced by others (O'Reilly, Aquino, and Skarlicki, 2016). When actors are involved in anger and frustration in injustice context, observers may have other considerations, because injustice poses a threat to observers' social identity (Tyler and Boeckmann, 1997); they need to psychologically distance themselves from the deviant offenders through some behavioral responses like punishment or prosocial tendency (Lotz et al., 2011), suggesting that the offenders are not representative of their group and the values held by the majority. In addition, observers may fear that injustice will one day be done to them if justice is not restored in a timely manner, especially if observers and actors belong to an organizational system. Therefore, it is much possible for observers to experience higher levels of negative other-focused moral emotions in the context of injustice.

Further, the high level of negative other-focused moral emotions among observers and actors in conditions of injustice provides strong empirical support for the inequality aversion model and also explains well why the experience of injustice is "hot and burning" (Li et al., 2022).

Nowadays, although we have already conducted a number of research in the field of exploring the interplay between emotions and theories of justice, we believe that we can still agree with the claim that this is a largely underresearched area (cf. Barclay, Skarlicki and Pugh, 2005, 629). This is surprising because: (i) justice and emotions are an important part of organizational life, characterizing and informing organizational processes as well as acting as communication systems that help individuals navigate through the basic problems that arise in social relations; (ii) and there is a strong theoretical association between (in)justice and emotion and from our perspective this is particularly evident in law and legal thinking. Weiss et al. (1999) argued that (in)justice could be understood as a special instance of more general appraisal models of emotion.

Simultaneously, let us not forget that the feeling of (in)justice is also an important evolutionary tool in combination with selected moral emotions. Particular attention was given to the relationship between the perception of injustice and the emotion of anger (Démuth, 2021, 2024). We should not underestimate the social dimension of anger. When we experience "egregious" injustice (individually, as a group, or as a society), we have a strong motivation to correct that injustice (even in cases where it may be strongly felt in third-party situations in which one has no stake). Racism, mass human rights violations, exploitation of others, and even ethnic cleansing or genocide can lead people who have no ties to the affected group to demand retaliatory or compensatory measures. We are now seeing more frequently emerging and visible global manifestations of anger toward certain negative phenomena. Thanks to social networks and easier communication across the globe, we are more likely to encounter angry resistance to the diverse problems that "plague" our lives – from various social issues such as discrimination based on gender, race, or sexual orientation; through political challenges such as the increasing radicalization and extremization of society; to the environmental difficulties of our planet. The various manifestations of opposition to state power are consequences of the evolutionarily proven mechanism of expressing anger as a means to change the behavior of those who have power but do not use it in accordance with our needs, desires or expectations. It is the moment of incongruence between the actions of those in power and our needs, desires, or expectations that is perceived as unfair from our perspective. In this, too, one can see significant aspects of the relationship between the feeling of injustice and the moral emotion of anger for our society.

As mentioned above, of course, many other moral emotions are also tied to the feeling of (in)justice (as a trigger). Emotions following justice-related events may color responses to specific event, to series of multiple events, and to entities as a whole; thus, emotional responses to justice event are a central part of justice experiences (Li et al., 2022). And compared to "basic" emotions, moral emotions involve substantial moral cognitive processing, e.g., why it is wrong to violate moral norms of justice (Malti and Ongley, 2014). It is the concept of moral emotions that can in many ways help us better understand how we behave in society. And despite the (also justified) criticism (see Démuth and Démuthová, 2023b, 22–26), we believe that moral emotions are critically important in understanding people's behavioral adherence to their moral standards. They provide the motivational force to do good and avoid doing bad (Tangney, Stuewig, and Mashek, 2007), and they can be perceived as states that occur when we perceive and evaluate a situation or a phenomenon within the dimensions of "desirable-undesirable" or "good-bad", not only from the perspective of the benefit to the individual but also considering the individual's coexistence with others (Démuth and Démuthová, 2023b, 23). And here the (often implicit) concept of (in)justice remains necessary.

Conclusion

In this study, we have attempted to demonstrate that the concept of (in)justice belongs among the essential concepts of architecture of human thought. We believe that it is clear that from our etymological, semantic, and contextual analysis, the notion of (in)justice represents a very complicated task. Justice and injustice are one of the most broadly based terms used in a language. It seems that although we intuitively grasp the meaning of the concept of (in)justice and some of its main semantic dimensions (and even in some cases selected disciplines work with a not precisely defined notion of (in)justice), once we try to understand it more precisely and with semantic clarity, the detailed and complete structure of the concept often escapes us. It is closely related to moral-juridical perception and a subsequent evaluation, which is affected by numerous factors. To identify the characteristics of both terms (justice and injustice) thus necessitates the consideration of a number of variables, which makes the creation of a complex notion complicated and ambiguous. However, we believe that this may not be an issue of a lack of objectivity, but rather in language users who focus on different basic dimensions of a concept of (in)justice, and thus on different semantic domains to which a particular user (and his/her chosen notion) relates.

This brings us to the conclusion that a closer understanding of the concept of (in)justice requires a detailed analysis of the more specific concepts and dimensions dealing with (in)justice and that "saturate" this concept in different cultural-linguistic contexts, through empirical analyses of the underlying (un)just concepts in different language users, as well as through an analysis of their semantic interrelationships with each other. The above might be a way to remove the ambiguity and semantic vagueness of the notion of (in)justice over time, but also to better understand how particular selected contexts (cultural/linguistic/national) influence our way of thinking about what is just and what is not.

It should be noted here, however, that there will (probably) always be a certain level of vagueness involved in the concept of (in)justice, and it is not necessary to view this as problematic in all circumstances. Of course, too much vagueness of concepts makes understanding impossible, and the primary function of language is also the need to communicate content in a way that is comprehensible. A certain degree of vagueness is fundamentally unavoidable in language, but this does not prevent us from possible knowledge and understanding (Démuth and Števček, 249-250) and the need to explore more closely the key concepts in human thought, which (in)justice undoubtedly is.

In this regard, the analysis of the concept of (in)justice, presented within this study, is an attempt in seeking to understand what (in)justice is and why it is important to focus on the concept as such, not just on particularistic issues related to what we experience as just or unjust in our lives. We believe that to understand (in)justice means to understand its terminology, evolutionary context, its etymology, and moral and social contingency. We have tried to focus on some interesting results of current research in this paper and to indicate the meanings of the concept of (in)justice for human morality and sociality.

References

Bambach, C. (2012). Heraclitean Justice between Heidegger and Nietzsche. In: Babich, B., Denker, A., Zaborowski, H. (eds.): *Heidegger & Nietzsche*. Leiden, The Netherlands: Brill, 235–245.

Bambach, C. (2021). Justice (Gerechtigkeit/Dikê). In: Wrathall M.A. (ed.), *The Cambridge Heidegger Lexicon*. Cambridge: Cambridge University Press, 440–442.

Barclay, L. J., Skarlicki, D. P., Pugh, S. D. (2005). Exploring the Role of Emotions in Injustice Perceptions and Retaliation. *Journal of Applied Psychology*, 90(4), 629–643.

Batka, Ľ. (2023). Spiritual and Theological Discernment of Good and Evil. In: Démuth, A., Démuthová, S. (eds.) *A Conceptual and Semantic Analysis of the Qualitative Domains of Aesthetic and Moral Motions: An Introduction*. Berlin : Peter Lang, 101–118.

Bárány, E. (2011). Spravodlivosť ako vzťahový pojem [Justice as a Relational Notion]. *Filozofia*, 66(9), 845–855.

Boatright, J. (2018). The History, Meaning, and Use of the Words Justice and Judge. *St. Mary's Law Journal*, 49(4), 727–748.

de Vaan, M. (2008). *Etymological Dictionary of Latin and the Other Italic Languages*. Leiden: Brill.

Démuth, A. (2021). Hnev ako sociálna a morálna emócia [Anger as a Social and Moral Emotion]. In: Szakács, A. et al. (eds.) *Bratislavské Právnické Fórum 2021* [Bratislava Legal Forum 2021]. Bratislava: Univerzita Komenského v Bratislave, Právnická fakulta, 23–30. Available at: https://www.researchgate.net/profile/Andrej-Demuth-2/publication/357061731_Hnev_ako_socialna_a_moralna_emocia/links/61ba20844b318a6970e30b3c/Hnev-ako-socialna-a-moralna-emocia.pdf (accessed on 25.05.2024).

Démuth, A., Števček, M. (2021). Defending Vagueness. *Filozofia* [Philosophy], 76(4), 237–251.

Démuth, A., Démuthová, S. (2023a). On the Indeterminacy of the Concept of Beauty and the Reasons for Its Use. *ESPES*, 12(1), 28–44.

Démuth, A., Démuthová, S. (2023b). An Introduction. In: Démuth, A., Démuthová, S. (eds.) *A Conceptual and Semantic Analysis of the Qualitative Domains of Aesthetic and Moral Motions: An Introduction*. Peter Lang, 7–38.

Démuth, A., Démuthová, S., Keceli, Y. (2023). On Some Etymological, Grammatical and Contextual Reasons for the Vagueness of the Concept of Beauty. In: Démuth, A., Démuthová, S. (eds.) *A Conceptual and Semantic Analysis of the Qualitative Domains of Aesthetic and Moral Motions: An Introduction*. Peter Lang, 39–56.

Démuth, A. (2024). *Anger as a Moral Emotion*. Berlin: Peter Lang.

Derksen, R. (2008). *Etymological Dictionary of the Slavic Inherited Lexicon*. Leiden, Boston, MA: Brill.

Doruľa, J. (1966). O niektorých starých slovenských slovách a právnych termínoch. [About Some Ancient Slovak Words and Legal Terms]. Československý terminologický časopis [*Czechoslovak Terminological Journal*], (5).

Doruľa, J. (1972). Slováci a ich reč (príspevok k starším dejinám slovenčiny) [Slovaks and Their Speech (Contribution to the Older History of the Slovak Language)]. *Jazykovedný časopis* [*The Linguistic Journal*], (2), 131–141.

Eisenberg, N. (2000). Emotion, regulation, and moral development. *Annual Review of Psychology*, 51(1), 665–697.

Gray, K., Wegner, D. M. (2011). Dimensions of Moral Emotions. *Emotion Review*, 3(3), 258–260.

Haidt, J. (2001). The Emotional Dog and Its Rational Tail: A Social Intuitionist Approach to Moral Judgment. *Psychological Review*, 108(4), 814–834.

Haidt, J. (2003). The Moral Emotions. In R. J. Davidson, K. R. Scherer, H. H. Goldsmith (eds.), *Handbook of Affective Sciences*. Oxford University Press, 852–870.

Haidt, J. (2012). *The Righteous Mind: Why Good People Are Divided by Politics and Religion*. New York: Pantheon Books.

Haidt, J. (2013). Moral Psychology and the Law: How Intuitions Drive Reasoning, Judgment, and the Search for Evidence. *Alabama Law Review*, 64(4), 867–880.

Halsey, C. S. (1889). *An Etymology of Latin and Greek*. Boston: Ginn, Heath. Available at: https://archive.org/details/etymologyoflatin00halsuoft/page/50/mode/2up?view=theater (accessed on 25.05.2024).

Hareli, S., Moran-Amir, O., David, S., Hess, U. (2013). Emotions as Signals of Normative Conduct. *Cognition & Emotion*, 27(8), 1395–1404.

Harper, D. (2024). *Online Etymology Dictionary*. Available at: https://www.etymonline.com/word/injustice#etymonline_v_9283 (accessed on 25.05.2024).

Heidegger, M. (2000). *Introduction to Metaphysics* (translated by G. Fried and R. Polt). Yale University Press.

Heinze, E. (2013). *The Concept of Injustice*. Abingdon, Routledge.

Homans, G. C. (1961). *Social Behavior: Its Elementary Forms*. New York: Harcourt, Brace & World.

Horberg, E., J., Oveis, C., Keltner, D. (2011). Emotions as Moral Amplifiers: An Appraisal Tendency Approach to the Influences of Distinct Emotions upon Moral Judgment. *Emotion Review*, 3(3), 237–244.

Hume, D. (2008). *A Treatise of Human Nature*. Wilmington: Nuvision Publications (Original Work Published 1739).

Gábriš, T., Jáger, R. (2016). *Najstaršie právo na Slovensku? pokus o rekonštrukciu predcyrilometodského normatívneho systému.* [The Most Ancient Law in Slovakia? An Attempt for Reconstruction of Pre-Cyrillomethodian Normative System]. Wolters Kluwer.

Kahneman, D., Klein, G. (2009). Conditions for Intuitive Expertise: A Failure to Disagree. *American Psychologist*, 64(6), 515–526.

Kahneman, D. (2011). *Thinking, Fast and Slow*. Farrar, Straus and Giroux.

Kelsen, H. (1933). *Ryzí nauka právní. Metoda a základní pojmy.* [Pure Theory of Law. Method and Basic Concepts]. Orbis.

Kišoňová, R. (2023). Considering the Emotion of Disgust in the Context of Terminology and Contemporary Literature. In: Démuth, A., Démuthová, S. (eds.) *A Conceptual and Semantic Analysis of the Qualitative Domains of Aesthetic and Moral Motions: An Introduction*. Peter Lang, 81–100.

Klabouch, J. (1995). Pluralistické výklady spravedlnosti [Pluralistic Interpretations of Justice]. *Právník*, 134(6), 558–562.

Klein, E. (1966). *A Comprehensive Etymological Dictionary of the English Language*. Elsevier Publishing Company.

Kluknavská, A. (2021). *Spravodlivosť v dejinách právneho, politického a sociálneho myslenia (od počiatku dejín myslenia po myšlienky K. Marxa)* [Justice in the History of Legal, Political and Social Thought (From the Beginning of the History of Thought to the Ideas of K. Marx)]. Univerzita Komenského, Právnická Fakulta.

Knapp, V. (1995). *Teorie práva* [Theory of Law]. C. H. Beck.

Kohlberg. L. (1969). Stage and Sequence: The Cognitive-Developmental Approach to Socialization. In: Goslin, D. A. (ed.). *Handbook of Socialisation Theory and Research*. Rand Mcnally, 347–480.

Kohlberg, L. (1973). The Claim to Moral Adequacy of a Highest Stage of Moral Judgment. *The Journal of Philosophy*, 70(18), 630–646.

Králik, Ľ. (2015). *Stručný etymologický slovník slovenčiny.* [A Brief Etymological Dictionary of Slovak]. Veda.

Krašovec, J. (2015). Semantics of the Concept of Justice and Its Literary Representations. *Bogoslovni vestnik*, 75(2), 313–322.

Lemm, V. (2013). Nietzsche and Heidegger on Justice. *Graduate Faculty Philosophy Journal*, 34(2), 439–455.

Li, X., Hou, M., He, Y., Ma, M. (2022). People Roar at the Sight of Injustice: Evidences from Moral Emotions. *Current Psychology*, Available at: https://doi.org/10.1007/s12144-022-04014-w (accessed on 25.12.2022).

Lotz, S., Okimoto, T., G., Schlösser, T., Fetchenhauer, D. (2011). Punitive Versus Compensatory Reactions to Injustice: Emotional Antecedents to Third-Party Interventions. *Journal of Experimental Social Psychology*, 47(2), 477–480.

Malti, T., Ongley, S. F. (2014). The Development of Moral Emotions and Moral Reasoning. In: M. Killen and J. G. Smetana (eds.), *Handbook of Moral Development* (pp. 163–183). Psychology Press.

Manly, J. M. (1916). *English Prose and Poetry (1137–1892)*. Boston, New York [etc.] Ginn and company. Available at: https://archive.org/details/cu31924013280189/page/n15/mode/2up (accessed on 25.05.2024).

Meteňkanyč, O. M. (2023). The relevance of legal intuitionism and selected moral emotions in legal thinking and decision-making processes. In: Démuth, A., Démuthová, S. (eds.) *A Conceptual and Semantic Analysis of the Qualitative Domains of Aesthetic and Moral Motions: An Introduction*. Peter Lang, 119–163.

Miller, D. (2021). Justice. In: Edward N. Zalta (ed.). *The Stanford Encyclopedia of Philosophy* (Fall 2021 Edition). available at: https://plato.stanford.edu/archives/fall2021/entries/justice/ (accessed on 25.12.2022).

Montanari, F. (2015). *The Brill Dictionary of Ancient Greek*. Leiden, Boston: Brill Hotei Publishing.

Mrva, M. (2018). Demokracia a právny štát [Democracy and the Rule of Law]. In: Kolektív autorov [Collective of Authors]. *Aktuálne otázky teórie práva* [Current Issues in the Theory of Law]. Wolters Kluwer, Univerzita Komenského, Právnická fakulta, 84–102.

Ondruš, Š. (2004). *Odtajnené trezory slov* [Declassified Safes of Words]. Vydavateľstvo Matice slovenskej.

Olivetti, E. (2024). *Online Latin Dictionary*. Available at: https://www.online-latin-dictionary.com/latin-english-dictionary.php?parola=ius (accessed on 25.05.2024).

O'Reilly, J., Aquino, K., Skarlicki, D. (2016). The Lives of Others: Third Parties' Responses to Others' Injustice. *Journal of Applied Psychology*, 101(2), 171–189.

Piaget, J. (1965). *The Moral Judgement of the Child* (Translated by M. Gabain). New York: Free Press (original work published 1932).

Plato. *Gorgias* (Translated by W.R.M. Lamb). Available at: https://www.perseus.tufts.edu/hopper/text?doc=urn:cts:greekLit:tlg0059.tlg023.perseus-eng1:469 (accessed on 25.05.2024).

Plato. *The Republic* (Translated by Benjamin Jowett). Available at: https://classics.mit.edu/Plato/republic.html (accessed on 25.05.2024).

Ramshorn, L. (1839). *Dictionary of Latin Synonyms*. Available at: https://archive.org/details/latin-synonyms-1839-03 (accessed on 25.05.2024).

Rejzek, J. (2001). *Český etymologický slovník*. [Czech Etymological Dictionary]. Leda.

Rudolph, U., Schulz, K., Tscharaktschiew, N. (2013). Moral Emotions: An Analysis Guided by Heider's Naive Action Analysis. *International Journal of Advances in Psychology*, 2(2), 69-92.

Rudolph, U., Tscharaktschiew, N. (2014). An Attributional Analysis of Moral Emotions: Naïve Scientists and Everyday Judges. *Emotion Review*, 6(4), 344-352.

Schmidtz, D. (2016). *Prvky spravodlivosti* [The Elements of Justice]. Dokořán.

Skeat, W. W. (1888). *An Etymological Dictionary of the English Language*. Oxford Clarendon Press. Available at: https://archive.org/details/etymologicaldict00skeauoft/page/n5/mode/2up (accessed on 25.05.2024).

Špaňár, J., Hrabovský, J. (2012). *Latinsko-slovenský, slovensko-latinský slovník*. [Latin-Slovak, Slovak-Latin Dictionary]. Slovenské pedagogické nakladateľstvo – Mladé letá.

Števček, M. (2018). Spravodlivosť, právo a slušnosť u Aristotela: krátka úvaha nad etikou Nikomachovou z pohľadu filozoficko-právneho. [Justice, Law and Decency in Aristotle: a Brief Reflection on the Ethics of Nicomacheus from a Philosophical-Legal Perspective]. In: *Ad iustitiam per ius* : pocta prof. PhDr. Jarmile Chovancovej, CSc. Wolters Kluwer, 2018, 37-57.

Tangney, P. J., Stuewig, J., Mashek, D. J. (2007). Moral Emotions and Moral Behavior. *Annual Review of Psychology*, 58(1), 345-372.

Tomsa, B. (2007). *Idea spravedlnosti a práva v řecké filosofii*. [The Idea of Justice and Law in Greek Philosophy]. Vydavatelství a nakladatelství Aleš Čeněk.

Tyler, T. R., Boeckmann, R. (1997). Three Strikes and You Are Out, but Why? The Psychology of Public Support for Punishing Rule Breakers. *Law and Society Review*, 31(2), 237-265.

Valpy, F. E. J. (1828). *An Etymological Dictionary of the Latin Language*. Available at: https://babel.hathitrust.org/cgi/pt?id=loc.ark:/13960/t8rb8cb9p&seq=226 (accessed on 25.05.2024).

Valpy, F. E. J. (1960). *The Etymology of the Words of the Greek Language*. Available at: https://archive.org/details/bub_gb_UYoCAAAAQAAJ/page/n43/mode/2up?view=theater (accessed on 25.05.2024).

Weinberger, O. (2010). *Inštitucionalizmus: Nová téoria konania, práva a demokracie* [Institutionalism: A New Theory of Action, Law and Democracy]. Kalligram.

Weinberger, O. (2017). *Norma a instituce – úvod do teorie práva* [Norms and Institutions – Introduction to the Theory of Law]. Aleš Čeněk.

Weiss, H., M., Suckow, K., Cropanzano, R. (1999). Effects of Justice Conditions on Discrete Emotions. *Journal of Applied Psychology*, 84(5), 786-794.

Weston, N. A. (2012). On Truth as Justice. In: Babich, B., Denker, A., Zaborowski, H. (eds.): *Heidegger & Nietzsche*. Leiden, The Netherlands: Brill, 441-455.

Cambridge Dictionary (2024). *Injustice*. Available at: https://dictionary.cambridge.org/thesaurus/injustice (accessed on 25.05.2024).

Cambridge Dictionary (2024). *Justice*. Available at: https://dictionary.cambridge.org/thesaurus/justice#google_vignette (accessed on 25.05.2024).

Collins Dictionary (2024). *Injustice*. Available at: https://www.collinsdictionary.com/dictionary/english-thesaurus/injustice#injustice__1 (accessed on 25.05.2024).

Dictionary of Slovak Synonyms (2004). *Nespravodlivosť*. Available at: https://slovnik.juls.savba.sk/?w=nespravodlivos%C5%A5&s=exact&c=Y6f4&cs=&d=kssj4&d=psp&d=sss&d=hssj# (accessed on 25.05.2024).

Dictionary of Slovak Synonyms (2004). *Spravodlivosť*. Available at: https://slovnik.juls.savba.sk/?w=spravodlivos%C5%A5&s=exact&c=043f&cs=&d=kssj4&d=psp&d=ogs&d=scs&d=sss&d=hssj# (accessed on 25.05.2024).

Merriam-Webster Dictionary (2024). *Injustice*. Available at: https://www.merriam-webster.com/thesaurus/injustice (accessed on 25.05.2024).

Oxford English Dictionary (2024). *Justice*. Available at: https://www.oed.com/dictionary/justice_n?tl=true&tab=meaning_and_use (accessed on 25.05.2024).

Oxford Dictionary (2024). *Injustice*. Available at: https://www.oxfordlearnersdictionaries.com/definition/english/injustice (accessed on 25.05.2024).

Oxford Latin Dictionary (1968). *Lexicon Universale Latinitatis*. Available at: https://archive.org/details/aa.-vv.-oxford-latin-dictionary-1968/page/984/mode/2up?view=theater (accessed on 25.05.2024).

Thesaurus (2024). *Injustice*. Available at: https://www.merriam-webster.com/thesaurus/injustice (accessed on 25.05.2024).

Thesaurus (2024). *Justice*. Available at: https://www.merriam-webster.com/thesaurus/justice (accessed on 25.05.2024).

Webster´s New Dictionary of Synonyms (1973). Springfield: G. & C. Merriam Co.

Outline of a Possible Mapping of Aesthetic and Moral Emotions
Summary or Conclusion?

Andrej Démuth

> *Attentive examination tends to generate questions rather than definitive answers. If the answers are definitive, it might indicate inattentiveness or a resignation from further exploration rather than complete knowledge.*

The intended goal of this collective monograph was to present some contemporary research on the cognitive nature of aesthetic and moral emotions within the humanities, in their interaction with cognitive science research. Additionally, we aimed to formulate the most unified and comprehensive theory of these emotions.

The primary question of our research was whether it is even necessary to speak of distinct aesthetic and moral emotions. Are they different from other emotions? If so, what distinguishes them? It seems that defining what constitutes moral or aesthetic emotions and whether there is even such a distinct category is highly problematic. The term "moral emotions" refers to a wide array of perceptions, feelings, emotional states, and emotions that arise in moral evaluation, judgment, decision-making, and action. What unites them are concepts like "good" or "evil", which themselves are very unclear, as evidenced by the history of philosophy and not entirely convincing attempts by various thinkers to define them. Nevertheless, it is evident that even without a clear and universally accepted definition, these concepts significantly influence our behavior.

Another significant problem is whether it is possible to "vertically"[23] separate bodily perceptions from feelings, impressions, and emotions. Are all examined aesthetic and moral emotions truly emotions, or are they rather fleeting and unclear feelings, or conversely, enduring passions or even attitudes? Is their nature bodily, occurring at the receptors, or is it rather an issue of consciousness, mind, or even values? Is there such a thing as a collective emotion, or is it just an unfortunate metaphor transferring meaning from the actual individual body to some imaginary collective body or society?

---

23 That is, from the bottom up.

This was also linked to another question regarding the subject of study. Are aesthetic emotions fundamentally different from moral ones? Do they have different natures or mechanisms? Why is it that in many languages we often interchange the evaluation of something as beautiful and good? Why do we say someone is acting badly if they are not nice to another person? Is it merely linguistic error or the imprecision of its users?

The presented studies suggest that both groups of emotions use very similar neurophysiological and neuroanatomical mechanisms for their emergence. We lean toward Damasio›s version of emotionality (Damasio, 1999), which understands emotions as reactive states of the organism to both internal and external stimuli. This explains why under the term "emotionality" or "emotional states", we can also refer to simple and immediate reactions of the organism, without any conscious or fully reflected personal stance – essentially more subconscious or not fully aware reactions. Similarly, however, this group of reactions also includes more complex perceptions, some of which still require taking a personal stance important to the individual, while for others, such intense subjective experience is characteristic and essential. Finally, we also tend to include the concept of emotionality reactions where the immediate affective response does not play the most crucial role and may not be outwardly noticeable. As a kind of cognitive set-up of the organism, it allows the individual to solve a given problem by taking a stance without showing a clear emotional expression. Ultimately, attitudes are characteristic in that they are products of previous personal or acquired experiences, not manifesting in emotional outbursts, but fundamentally influencing our actions.

Why then do we possess emotionality and emotional states if they are so diverse and seemingly contradictory? It seems, and here we must agree with Owen Flanagan (Flanagan, 2021), that it is an adaptive reaction of the organism, enabling it to respond to stimuli in some effective way. If a given reaction allows the organism to survive, its pattern becomes entrenched and survives with its carrier. If the reaction is inappropriate and does not provide evolutionary advantages, its carrier perishes. The role of emotions is primarily to inform the organism about the presence of certain stimuli in the individual›s internal or external environment. This happens in such a way that the organism responds specifically to these stimuli. Where it is unnecessary (for instance, because the conditions in the environment do not change significantly over time), the organism adopts fully automatic reactions – reflexes, instincts, etc. In such cases, it is not necessary to take specific stances. In fact, as in the case of a burn, it would be counterproductive to react only after fully realizing the structural damage to the tissue caused by burning. Automatism allows the organism to save time and energy, and because it is effective, this form of behavior has settled in our repertoire of reactions as efficient. Where it was not effective, we changed it, or its carriers became extinct.

However, where there is no single definitively correct answer, or where, given the complexity or variability of conditions, a particular reaction can be both good and bad (in the context of its long-term consequences), it is more advantageous to inform the organism about the presence of such stimuli and conditions so that it can efficiently seek the best possible reaction. An example might be the acquired ability to respond to glucose intake with pleasant feelings, but also the ability to avoid excessive consumption, for instance, for health reasons. Therefore, in addition to unconscious or instinctive reactions, we also possess behaviors that require the possibility of control, veto, or direction, and even those that by their very nature assume rational (i.e., as minimally emotionally blinded as possible) and planned behavior.

The thesis we present here is the belief that most feelings and emotions have arisen as adaptive reactions to the presence of specific – important for the organism – stimuli and at the same time, they serve to support the organism in responding to these stimuli in an evolutionarily appropriate manner (Démuthová, 2019).

For emotions to function as responses to specific stimuli, it is necessary for the organism to be sensitive to those stimuli. In the case of the aforementioned sugar (glucose), discovering and consuming it provided the individual with the advantage of a quickly and easily digestible energy source, hence leading to its pursuit. The impetus for seeking such a source was its easy utilization, which did not burden the body with strenuous food acquisition and difficult digestion.[24] Therefore, such behavior was rewarded with pleasant feelings, contrasting with those that emerged, for

---

24 For example, compared to fats.

instance, from the consumption of alkaloids. Similarly, many feelings and emotions can be considered mechanisms that motivate the organism to respond to stimuli in either a desirable or undesirable way, akin to rewards and punishments.

From a neurophysiological and neuroanatomical perspective, ancient brain structures, such as the limbic system, the amygdala (which is part of it), and the reward circuit play a key role in emotionality. It appears that both types of emotional states (aesthetic and moral emotions) arose for very similar purposes. Their role is to support a certain kind of behavior in response to specific conditions in the internal or external environment. However, there is indeed a difference between them. Aesthetic emotions often seem to be more rigidly linked to ancient evolutionary heritage (e.g., physical attractiveness being an indicator of robust and suitable genes),[25] whereas moral emotions are more frequently shaped by upbringing or other personally acquired experiences. While pleasant feelings from the beauty of a figure or landscape often have evolutionary roots, similar to physical disgust, anger is more problematic, and guilt and injustice clearly refer to personal experience and cultural context. This is because moral emotions more frequently respond to very complex social situations. These can have immediate visible consequences or long-term ones depending on many variables. Therefore, it is necessary to calculate and consider the possible relatively rapid changes in the environment. This is particularly evidenced by the connection between moral affectivity and the activity of the prefrontal cortex and frontal lobes, which are responsible for planning and focused attention. Thus, it is not about automated reactions but rather complex computational activity aimed at evaluating multiple possible scenarios. This is more evident in moral judgment. Moral emotions take into account the variability of the social environment, while in the search for suitable genes (predominantly aesthetic emotions), the environmental circumstances determining our taste change very slowly. In other words, natural and cultural evolution do not progress at the same pace; their clocks are not synchronized.

---

[25] Although a large number of aesthetic feelings and emotions are also shaped by individual experience and upbringing – consider fashion, art, etc.

As Soren Kierkegaard (Kierkegaard, 1986) demonstrated, our ability to feel guilt emerges only after the awakening of the sleeping spirit, that is, after eating from the tree of knowledge. Similarly, Ľubomír Batka, along with Heidegger and Ricoeur, thematizes the primordiality of guilt before innocence. Humans are not born with the awareness of guilt; it is gradually discovered, usually after recognizing the discrepancy between what should have been done and what was actually done. Guilt and the sense of injustice are primarily matters of upbringing. However, beauty is different. Even young children feel pleasant sensations from certain stimuli. They look longer at faces deemed beautiful in their environment and react with displeasure to ugliness or unpleasant stimuli. What is pleasant to us simply appeals to us, and we consider it good in a certain way. Although our taste evolves over time, it seems we are born with a sensitivity to certain kinds of beauty.

Despite their differences, moral emotions have similar evolutionary roots and functions. They encourage us to do what we consider appropriate and warn against what we have learned to be wrong. The feelings of beauty and goodness are evolutionarily similar, as are the terms we use to describe them.

In the history of psychology, we find several theories that believe in the discreteness of individual emotions. Some thinkers assert that we have five, six, or another number of basic emotions, fundamentally different in their experience, function, and manifestations. For these states, we have specific terms and labels in our language. Other emotions (secondary) are supposedly derived from them and are their derivatives. Although we sometimes have specific conceptual schemes, terms, or labels for them, their boundaries are not as sharp or clear, and we sometimes struggle to conceptually grasp or name a specific emotional state. Furthermore, different languages map the emotional reality differently. Some languages have specific terms for concepts like "Schadenfreude", while others do not and use descriptive expressions. Different languages, therefore, seem to act merely as various types of classification and representation of experienced reality, raising the question of the realism and constructivism of emotions. Another issue with the realist belief in basic emotions is whether and how emotional mixing is possible, or whether we can identify the pure, primary, and original emotions in their uncontaminated form if they are to have discrete boundaries.

Contrarily, there is an approach that believes emotions are more continuous, or rather, multidimensional objects differing in the degree of saturation of various dimensions of their experience. Such concepts might better explain the full variability of our feelings and emotions. Even here, we encounter the problem of the boundaries of individual emotions and the realism and constructivism issue – whether emotions exist in reality or are merely social constructs of language.

In this work, we have attempted to suggest possibilities for bridging both approaches. The advantage of a discrete understanding of emotions lies in their non-arbitrary labeling, which prompts realism – the belief that universal basic emotional states exist and have nearly identical conceptual schemes across different languages, despite differing terminological captures. This ancient philosophical-psychological doctrine is supported by some neurophysiological findings. Wang and colleagues (Wang, Pereira 2016; Gu et al. 2018; Gu et al. 2019a, 2019b; Jiang et al. 2022) have identified a specific neuromodulator for each basic emotion. Differences in neuromodulators thus cause differences in emotions and subsequently their naming. However, the same Wang and Pereira (Wang, Pereira, 2016) also present a semantic model allowing the application of a continuous understanding of emotions. The combination of various neuromodulators results in our frequently encountering mixed derivatives of feelings in everyday experience rather than their pure forms.

Despite possible shortcomings of his original approach (a planar understanding of emotionality and the antagonistic action of neuromodulators such as ACH vs. NE and dopamine vs. serotonin), this model, when corrected to a spatial multidimensional model, better explains the complexities and interrelations of individual emotions based on the number and degree of involved neuromodulators. Emotions can thus be understood as fluidly transitioning and differing multidimensional objects, primarily varying in the degree of saturation of individual (semantic) dimensions. The problem of this approach is not why feelings can mix, but rather their naming.

A continuous model of emotions must elucidate the reasons why we label one semantic domain in a certain way and another differently. To address this issue, we can utilize Gärdenfors' model of the geometry of thought and semantic spaces. Peter Gärdenfors posits that for important areas of our lives, we possess concepts and terms that map the mental world we experience and navigate. This semantic world is similar to (or strives to closely resemble) the real physical space it describes, and thus also the mental world constituted by physical sensations. According to Gärdenfors, the semantic world can be described through conceptual spaces, which are akin to geometrical or physical spaces, being representations based on a certain number of quality dimensions. "The primary function of quality dimensions is to represent different 'qualities' of objects" (Gärdenfors 2015, p. 23). These qualities can be natural (innate or developed early on). Such qualities are to some extent hardwired into our nervous system.[26] Other dimensions can be culturally dependent. Emotional concepts, or concepts designating emotions, then represent (natural) concepts whose function is to label various mental objects (feelings, states, emotions, passions, attitudes) based on their fundamental quality dimensions. Thus, they represent conceptual spaces or regions. Their peculiarity is that they denote convex regions of the given mental space. "A convex region is characterized by the criterion that for any pair of points v1 and v2 in the region, all points between v1 and v2 are also part of the region. The reason for this criterion is that if some objects located at v1 and v2 in relation to a certain quality dimension (or several dimensions) both fall under concept C, then any object situated between v1 and v2 on the given quality dimension(s) will also fall under concept C" (Gärdenfors 2015, p. 34). This means that every point in a given area not only has proximity to the center of the area but all its semantic derivatives also belong to that area. In such a model, the feeling of anger would represent the entire area of the mental space created by anger and its derivatives (where pure anger is at the center of this area, and the derivatives extend toward other feelings according to the degree and intensity of saturation of those emotions). If a given feeling is closer to the center of another feeling, it is semantically subsumed by it (identified more as this other feeling (e.g., sadness)

---

26 Like hardwired connections in a computer. Gärdenfors uses the English term "hardwired" (Gärdenfors 2004).

rather than anger). For important types of emotions (their prototypes), we have individual central (focal) concepts. Either they represent the actual focal point of the entire given conceptual convex region or they are a prototype, meaning a construct of how the given emotion should appear. These denote the entire area of those feelings according to their focal points. This means that for some very complex feelings, we can have a wealth of synonymous or semantically related terms (e.g., rage, hatred, aggression, defiance...), which fall under a broader central (focal) concept (e.g., anger). If an emotion lies more within the scope of another focal point, we label it with the focal concept of that area (if the feeling has more sadness than anger, we label it as sadness). Thus, the semantic areas of individual emotions can be further subdivided into smaller subspaces according to the specificity and interplay of their individual dimensions.

The use of Gärdenfors› model allows for the semantic (conceptual) mapping of individual mental spaces we navigate. This enables a subject to convey to another what they are experiencing by naming the given semantic area and indicating the more precise conceptual topography of that semantic space. Although it might be true, as Nagel suggests, that the qualities of our feelings as qualia are unique and irreducible due to the uniqueness of each organism and the unrepeatable composition of its receptors or brain, this approach allows at least a rough mapping of the mental world, thereby facilitating the meeting of two minds. This encounter and its motivations are driven primarily by pragmatic reasons.

As with other concepts, when it comes to the linguistic capture of emotional states, what motivates us is primarily cooperation or the ability to predict the behavior of others. Hence, for emotional states that occur frequently or are important, we usually have a richer vocabulary, and their semantic areas are more accurately and thoroughly mapped. Where this is not crucial for sharing, we do not concern ourselves as much with precision of terms.

Gärdenfors› model provides a framework for potentially capturing the mapping of mental semantic spaces. Its significant challenge, however, lies in determining the individual semantic dimensions of a given semantic space. Wang›s realistic solution was simple – it relied on different neuromodulators. But how does this apply to semantic dimensions?

Gärdenfors explains his model using colors, based on the existence of three fundamental characteristics of all colors: hue, brightness, and saturation. Do we have such uniform dimensions for all emotional states?

Our psycholinguistic research relied primarily on the analysis of synonyms and connotations that best capture the scope and breadth of a given semantic area of a mental space. By sorting and clustering these associations, the diversity of dimensions associated with these words in the minds of their users can be mapped. However, it turned out that the most direct way to uncover the individual dimensions of terms describing emotions is through the examination of their antonyms. Antonyms can indicate the basic (albeit partial) dimensions in which a word is used. Their set thus well indicates the different semantic areas in which the original word is used. This can be empirically investigated even with ordinary (non-psychologically trained) users to discover with what and how these terms are associated in their everyday language. This can also be done through a conceptual analysis of dictionary definitions of individual terms – their definitions, synonyms, etc., among trained experts or scientists. This way, the objective meaning of terms and their scope in a given language can be studied. However, we were more interested in what a given emotion or its designation means to each individual. Using the traditional semantic differential, we attempted to understand the subjective (connotative) meanings of individual words and compare their perceptions across different groups (by gender, age, etc.).[27] A significant part of the research focused on the subjective understanding of the emotions we experience. This focus arises not only because we believe that subjective experience precedes any objective theory or theory of meaning. Emotions are felt "on" or under our own skin. They are primarily messages and signals for us. Only subsequently, after considering the specifics of each user, can we contemplate their objective meaning or role. Such contemplation can then help us understand what and why we actually experience. This was the goal of our research.

We reflected on why we like what we like, the essence of admiration or disgust, and why we get angry. We explored guilt and

---

27 See: Démuth, Démuthová, Keceli, 2022a; Démuth, Démuthová, Keceli, 2022b.

its functions, considering where and why the feeling of injustice arises and our desire for its rectification. Not all investigations were completed. Perhaps it is beyond our capabilities or even our task. Rather, we aimed to contribute to the growing research on aesthetic and moral emotionality. We hoped to inspire the reader to pay closer attention to their own feelings. Lastly, we aimed to highlight that emotionality is not irrationality in the sense of lacking a rational basis or potential for rational understanding and explanation. It is rather an alternative rationality – rationality of a different nature, not always accessible to conscious awareness. The apparent irrationality of feelings and emotions is an illusion born of misunderstanding or superficial perspective. The fact that we sometimes do not perceive the rational reasons and causes does not mean they do not exist or are irrational. On the contrary, it might be a challenge to thematize the states in which we exist for most of our lives, almost dominantly (even if we might think they are insignificant). It is a challenge not to prioritize the idea of a rational and disembodied self over the daily experienced "here and now" of our mind and body.[28] After all, we are not rational systems that have emotions but rather emotional systems that sometimes behave rationally.

References

Batka, Ľ. (2024). Guilt. Persons in Web of Guilt. Guilt in Net of Interpretations. (in this volume).

Damasio, A. (1999). *The Feeling of What Happens: Body, Emotion and the Making of Consciousness*. Vintage.

Démuth A., Démuthová S. & Keçeli Y. (2022a). A Semantic Analysis of the Concept of Beauty (Güzellik) in Turkish Language: Mapping the Semantic Domains. *Frontiers in Communication*. 7:797316. doi: 10.3389/fcomm.2022.797316

Démuth, A., Démuthová, S., Keceli, Y. (2022b): A Semantic Analysis of the Concept of Anger and Its Connotations in the Turkish Language. Любословие. 22, 111–127.

Démuthová, S. (2019). Krása v kontexte evolučných prístupov [Beauty in the Context of Evolutionary Approaches] *Filosofický časopis, 67*(4), 591–603.

---

28 Whatever the two terms may be intended to mean.

Flanagan, O. (2021). *How to Do Things with Emotions*. Princeton University Press.

Gärdenfors, P. (2004). Conceptual Spaces as a Framework for Knowledge Representation. *Behavioral and Brain Sciences*, 27(3), 403. https://doi.org/10.1017/S0140525X04280098

Gärdenfors, P. (2015). Konceptuálne priestory [Conceptual Spaces]. In: Démuth, A. (ed.). *Geometrizovanie myslenia. Vybrané štúdie ku kognitívnej sémantike. [Geometrization of thinking. selected studies on cognitive semantics.]* (pp. 21–45): Schola Philosophica.

Gu, S., Gao, M., Yan, Y., Wang, F., Tang, Y. Y., & Huang, J. H. (2018). The Neural Mechanism Underlying Cognitive and Emotional Processes in Creativity. *Frontiers in Psychology*, 9, 1924. https://doi.org/10.3389/fpsyg.2018.01924.

Gu, S., Wang, F., Cao, C., Wu, E., Tang, Y. Y., & Huang, J. H. (2019a). An Integrative Way for Studying Neural Basis of Basic Emotions with fMRI. *Frontiers in Neuroscience*, 13, 628. https://doi.org/10.3389/fnins.2019.00628.

Gu, S., Wang, F., Patel, N. P., Bourgeois, J. A., & Huang, J. H. (2019b). A Model for Basic Emotions Using Observations of Behavior. *Drosophila. Frontiers in Psychology*, 10, 781. https://doi.org/10.3389/fpsyg.2019.00781.

Jiang, Y., Zou, D., Li, Y., Gu, S., Dong, J., Ma, X., Xu, S., Wang, F., & Huang, J. H. (2022). Monoamine Neurotransmitters Control Basic Emotions and Affect Major Depressive Disorders. *Pharmaceuticals (Basel, Switzerland)*, 15(10), 1203. https://doi.org/10.3390/ph15101203.

Kierkegaard, S., A. (1986). *Fear and Trembling*. Penguin Classics.

Wang, F., & Pereira, A. (2016). Neuromodulation, Emotional Feelings and Affective Disorders. *Mens Sana Monographs*, 14(1), 5–29. https://doi.org/10.4103/0973-1229.154533.

Notes on Contributors

Ľubomír Batka is Professor at the Department of Theory of Law and Philosophy of Law, Faculty of Law, and Comenius University in Bratislava. He earned his PhD at Eberhard-Karls Universität in Tübingen, in the field of Protestant Theology and habilitated at Comenius University in Bratislava. He was visiting Fellow at Leibniz Institute for European History in Mainz. Currently, he works and publishes in ethics and bioethics.
https://orcid.org/0000-0002-4128-4260

Andrej Démuth studied philosophy and psychology. He is Professor of Philosophy and Head of the Center for Cognitive Studies at the Department of Theory of Law and Philosophy of Law, Faculty of Law, Comenius University in Bratislava. He is the author of many books and articles on cognition and the relationship between reflected and non-reflected knowledge, and he regularly gives invited lectures at universities in Slovakia and abroad. His research focuses on modern philosophy, epistemology, and cognitive studies.
https://orcid.org/0000-0003-3133-2908

Slávka Démuthová is Professor of Psychology and Head of the Centre for the Psychological Counselling and Research at the Faculty of Arts, University of Ss. Cyril and Methodius in Trnava, Slovakia. Her professional orientation focuses on the developmental problems of children and youth as well as on the biological/evolutionary explanations of human behavior. She is an author of several monographs and scientific articles, and regularly gives invited lectures at universities abroad (Edinburgh, Brno, Prague, Warsaw, and Ljubljana).
https://orcid.org/0000-0003-1879-6871

Renáta Kišoňová studied philosophy at Trnava University. She works as Lecturer at the Department of Theory of Law and Philosophy of Law, Faculty of Law, Comenius University in Bratislava. Her research interests include the problems of cognitive aesthetics, mainly the issue of facial and portrait´s perception. She has also published a monograph "Faces of a face. Portraiture as a means of representing faces". Currently, she focuses on the problem of social and aesthetical emotions of disgust and admiration.
https://orcid.org/0000-0002-3869-0065

Olexij M. Meteňkanyč studied law and philosophy. He is Assistant Professor at the Department of Theory of Law and Philosophy of Law, Faculty of Law, Comenius University in Bratislava. He is the author and co-author of numerous scientific articles and textbooks, and in his academic activities, he not only addresses general theoretical, legal-philosophical and ethical issues but also focuses specifically on the topic of justice, both at the legal-philosophical level (in particular, in the recent debates between representatives of iusnaturalism and iuspositivism) and in the human rights sphere (especially the protection of the human rights of minorities). He regularly participates in national and international conferences, seminars, and workshops.
https://orcid.org/0000-0002-5894-0906

www.ingramcontent.com/pod-product-compliance
Ingram Content Group UK Ltd.
Pitfield, Milton Keynes, MK11 3LW, UK
UKHW021845140426
5217IPUK00022B/1598